Evidence-Based Veterinary Medicine for the Bovine Veterinarian

Guest Editors

SÉBASTIEN BUCZINSKI, Dr Vét, DÉS, MSc
JEAN-MICHEL VANDEWEERD, DMV, MS

VETERINARY CLINICS OF NORTH AMERICA: FOOD ANIMAL PRACTICE

www.vetfood.theclinics.com

Consulting Editor
ROBERT A. SMITH, DVM, MS

March 2012 • Volume 28 • Number 1

SAUNDERS an imprint of ELSEVIER, Inc.

W.B. SAUNDERS COMPANY
A Division of Elsevier Inc.

1600 John F. Kennedy Boulevard • Suite 1800 • Philadelphia, PA 19103-2899

http://www.vetfood.theclinics.com

VETERINARY CLINICS OF NORTH AMERICA: FOOD ANIMAL PRACTICE Volume 28, Number 1
March 2012 ISSN 0749-0720, ISBN-13: 978-1-4557-3953-0

Editor: John Vassallo; j.vassallo@elsevier.com
Developmental Editor: Teia Stone

Veterinary Clinics of North America: Food Animal Practice (ISSN 0749-0720) is published in March, July, and November by Elsevier Inc., 360 Park Avenue South, New York, NY 10010-1710. Subscription prices are $215.00 per year (domestic individuals), $296.00 per year (domestic institutions), $100.00 per year (domestic students/ residents), $243.00 per year (Canadian individuals), $387.00 per year (Canadian institutions), $307.00 per year (international individuals), $387.00 per year (international institutions), and $153.00 per year (international and Canadian students/ residents). To receive student/resident rate, orders must be accompained by name of affiliated institution, date of term, and the signature of program/residency coordinator on institution letterhead. *Clinics* subscription prices. All prices are subject to change without notice. **POSTMASTER:** Send address changes to *Veterinary Clinics of North America: Food Animal Practice,* Elsevier Health Sciences Division, Subscription Customer Service, 3251 Riverport Lane, Maryland Heights, MO 63043. Customer Service (orders, claims, online, change of address): Elsevier Health Sciences Division, Subscription Customer Service, 3251 Riverport Lane, Maryland Heights, MO 63043. Tel: 1-800-654-2452 (U.S. and Canada); 314-447-8871 (ouside U.S. and Canada). Fax: 314-447-8029. E-mail: journalscustomerservice-usa@elsevier.com (for print support); journalsonlinesupport-usa@elsevier.com (for online support).

Reprints. For copies of 100 or more, of articles in this publication, please contact the Commercial Reprints Department, Elsevier Inc., 360 Park Avenue South, New York, NY 10010-1710. Tel.: 212-633-3812; Fax: 212-462-1935; E-mail: reprints@elsevier.com.

Veterinary Clinics of North America: Food Animal Practice is covered in *Current Contents/Agriculture, Biology and Environmental Sciences, MEDLINE/PubMed (Index Medicus),* and *Excerpta Medica.*

Printed and bound by CPI Group (UK) Ltd, Croydon, CR0 4YY
Transferred to Digital Print 2011

Contributors

CONSULTING EDITOR

ROBERT A. SMITH, DVM, MS
Diplomate, American Board of Veterinary Practitioners; Veterinary Research and Consulting Services, LLC, Greeley, Colorado

GUEST EDITORS

SÉBASTIEN BUCZINSKI, Dr Vét, DÉS, MSc
Diplomate, American College of Veterinary Internal Medicine; Département des Sciences Cliniques, Faculté de Médecine Vétérinaire, St-Hyacinthe, Université de Montréal, Québec, Canada

JEAN-MICHEL VANDEWEERD, DMV, MS, Cert ES (soft tissue)
Diplomate, European College of Veterinary Surgeons; Integrated Veterinary Research Unit - Namur Research Institute for Life Sciences, Department of Veterinary Medicine, Faculty of Sciences, University of Namur, Namur, Belgium

AUTHORS

MIKE APLEY, DVM, PhD
Diplomate, American College of Veterinary Clinical Pharmacology; Department of Clinical Sciences, College of Veterinary Medicine, Kansas State University, Manhattan, Kansas

AUBREY N. BAIRD, MS, DVM
Diplomate, American College of Veterinary Surgeons; Associate Professor, Department of Veterinary Clinical Sciences, Purdue University, West Lafayette, Indiana

SÉBASTIEN BUCZINSKI, Dr Vét, DÉS, MSc
Diplomate, American College of Veterinary Internal Medicine; Département des Sciences Cliniques, Faculté de Médecine Vétérinaire, St-Hyacinthe, Université de Montréal, Québec, Canada

PETER CLEGG, VetMB, MA, PhD
Department of Veterinary Clinical Science and Husbandry, University of Liverpool, Leahurst, Neston, Cheshire, United Kingdom

PETER D. CONSTABLE, BVSc(Hons), MS, PhD
Diplomate, American College of Veterinary Internal Medicine; Diplomate, American College of Veterinary Nutrition; Professor and Head, Department of Veterinary Clinical Sciences, Purdue University, West Lafayette, Indiana

TODD F. DUFFIELD, DVM, DVSc
Professor of Ruminant Health Management, Department of Population Medicine, Ontario Veterinary College, University of Guelph, Guelph, Ontario, Canada

DAVID FRANCOZ, DMV, DÉS, MSc
Département des Sciences Cliniques, Faculté de Médecine Vétérinaire, St-Hyacinthe, Université de Montréal, Québec, Canada

PASCAL GUSTIN, DMV, PhD
Diplomate, European College for Veterinary Toxicology; Department of Functionnal Sciences, Faculty of Veterinary Medicine, University of Liège, Liège, Belgium

V. HOUGARDY, BSc
CHR–Site de La Citadelle, University of Liège, Liège, Belgium

MARIE-FRANCE HUMBLET, DMV, MSc, PhD
Research Unit in Epidemiology and Risk Analysis Applied to Veterinary Sciences (UREAR), Department of Infectious and Parasitic Diseases, Faculty of Veterinary Medicine, University of Liège, Liège, Belgium

GREG KEEFE, DVM, MSc, MBA
Professor, Department of Health Management, Atlantic Veterinary College, University of Prince Edward Island, Prince Edward Island, Canada

R.L. LARSON, DVM, PhD
Diplomate, American College of Theriogenologists; Diplomate, American College of Veterinary Preventive Medicine - Epidemiology; Professor, Coleman Chair Food Animal Production Medicine, Department of Clinical Sciences, College of Veterinary Medicine, Kansas State University, Manhattan, Kansas

IAN J. LEAN, BVSc, PhD, MACVSc
Managing Director, SBScibus, Camden, New South Wales, Australia

REJEAN C. LEFEBVRE, DMV, PhD
Diplomate, American College of Theriogenologists; Département des Sciences Cliniques, Faculté de Médecine Vétérinaire, St-Hyacinthe, Université de Montréal, Québec, Canada

LUDOVIC MARTINELLE, DMV, MSc
Research Unit in Epidemiology and Risk Analysis Applied to Veterinary Sciences (UREAR), Department of Infectious and Parasitic Diseases, Faculty of Veterinary Medicine, University of Liège, Liège, Belgium

MOHAMMAD NOURI, DVM, PhD
Professor, Department of Clinical Sciences, College of Veterinary Medicine, Shahid Chamran University, Ahvaz, Iran

REBECCA PORTER, DMV, MSc, PhD
Research Unit in Epidemiology and Risk Analysis Applied to Veterinary Sciences (UREAR), Department of Infectious and Parasitic Diseases, Faculty of Veterinary Medicine, University of Liège, Liège, Belgium

AHMAD RABIEE, DVM, PhD
Research Director, SBScibus, Camden, New South Wales, Australia

JEAN-PHILIPPE ROY, DVM, MSc
Diplomate, European College of Bovine Health Management; Professor, Département des Sciences Cliniques, Faculté de Médecine Vétérinaire, St-Hyacinthe, Université de Montréal, Québec, Canada

CLAUDE SAEGERMAN, DMV, MSc, PhD
Diplomate, European College of Veterinary Public Health; Professor and Head of Department, Research Unit in Epidemiology and Risk Analysis Applied to Veterinary Sciences (UREAR), Department of Infectious and Parasitic Diseases, Faculty of Veterinary Medicine, University of Liège, Liège, Belgium

ISMAIL SEN, DVM, PhD
Professor, Department of Internal Medicine, Faculty of Veterinary Medicine, University of Selcuk, Konya, Turkey

D.L. STEP, DVM
Diplomate, American College of Veterinary Internal Medicine; Professor, Department of Veterinary Clinical Sciences, Center for Veterinary Health Sciences, Oklahoma State University, Stillwater, Oklahoma

ANGELIKA E. STOCK, DMV, PhD
Diplomate, American College of Theriogenologists; Département des Sciences Cliniques, Faculté de Médecine Vétérinaire, St-Hyacinthe, Université de Montréal, Québec, Canada

FRANCISCO A. UZAL, DVM, MSc, PhD
Diplomate, American College of Veterinary Pathologists; Professor of Diagnostic Pathology, California Animal Health and Food Safety, San Bernardino Branch, University of California, Davis, San Bernardino, California

JEAN-MICHEL VANDEWEERD, DMV, MS, Cert ES (soft tissue)
Diplomate, European College of Veterinary Surgeons; Integrated Veterinary Research Unit - Namur Research Institute for Life Sciences, Department of Veterinary Medicine, Faculty of Sciences, University of Namur, Namur, Belgium

THOMAS WITTEK, Dr. habil
Diplomate, European College of Bovine Health Management; Professor, Department for Farm Animals and Veterinary Public Health, University of Veterinary Medicine Vienna, Vienna, Austria

GINA ZANELLA, DMV, MSc, PhD
Epidemiology Unit, Animal Health Laboratory, ANSES, Maisons-Alfort Cedex, France

Contents

Preface: Evidence-Based Veterinary Medicine **xiii**

Sébastien Buczinski and Jean-Michel Vandeweerd

How Can Veterinarians Base Their Medical Decisions on the Best Available Scientific Evidence? **1**

Jean-Michel Vandeweerd, Peter Clegg, and Sébastien Buczinski

With the advent of a One World-One Health concept, veterinarians will play a central role, at the level of trading zones (such as the European Union), countries, food production farms, and individual animals. They will be mandated to produce, interpret, communicate, and apply scientific information in the best possible way to make informed decisions and take adequate actions. The principles of evidence-based medicine will help the accomplishment of this mission. However, for the moment, we may still have the impression of two separate worlds, the academic research on one side and the reality of practice on the other side, and there is a need to join them.

Using Systematic Reviews to Critically Appraise the Scientific Information for the Bovine Veterinarian **13**

Jean-Michel Vandeweerd, Peter Clegg, V. Hougardy, and Sébastien Buczinski

Bovine veterinarians need to base their clinical decisions on the best scientific evidence. Due to lack of time, the relevant information should be available in a structured and summarized publication, such as systematic reviews. The results and the discussion should be reported in a practical and useful way. A structured abstract helps the busy practitioner to have a quick look on the evidence gained by this approach. There is a lack of studies in many areas of ruminant health compared with human health. Although this can be perceived as a limitation, veterinarians and scientists should design strategies to develop more systematic reviews.

Evidence Related to the Use of Ancillary Drugs in Bovine Respiratory Disease (Anti-Inflammatory and Others): Are They Justified or Not? **23**

David Francoz, Sébastien Buczinski, and Mike Apley

The therapeutic approach for bovine respiratory disease (BRD) includes antimicrobial treatment due to the frequent implication of bacteria. The data concerning the use of ancillary drugs (such as anti-inflammatory drugs or immunomodulators) are scant and often are based on experimental models of BRD. The effect of NSAIDs on pulmonary lesions, despite appearing beneficial, remains to be confirmed in well-designed, long-term trials. The impact on weight gain is inconsistent in these studies. This review emphasized the need for articles concerning clinical trials to

Therapeutic Efficiency of Antibiotics and Prostaglandin $F_{2\alpha}$ in Postpartum Dairy Cows with Clinical Endometritis: An Evidence-Based Evaluation **79**

Rejean C. Lefebvre and Angelika E. Stock

The occurrence of vaginal discharge in postpartum dairy cows is generally diagnosed as clinical endometritis. This uterine condition is associated with reduced fertility and economic loss for the dairy industry. Therapeutic approaches include the systemic or intrauterine application of antibiotics or the injection of prostaglandin $F_{2\alpha}$ and analogues to cause luteolysis and uterine contractions to evacuate the infected content. The treatment of clinical endometritis remains a subject of considerable controversy in the literature. Better understanding of the reproductive biology of normal versus abnormal uterine involution and immune mechanisms will allow more efficient diagnostic methods and a more efficient therapeutic approach.

Evidence-Based Effectiveness of Vaccination Against *Mannheimia haemolytica, Pasteurella multocida,* and *Histophilus somni* in Feedlot Cattle for Mitigating the Incidence and Effect of Bovine Respiratory Disease Complex **97**

R.L. Larson and D.L. Step

Bovine respiratory disease complex is the leading cause of morbidity and mortality in feedlot cattle. A number of vaccines against bacterial respiratory pathogens are commercially available and researchers have studied their impact on morbidity, mortality, and other disease outcome measures in feedlot cattle. A systematic review will provide veterinarians with a rigorous and transparent evaluation of the published literature to estimate the extent of vaccine effect. Unfortunately, the published body of evidence does not provide a consistent estimate of the direction and magnitude of effectiveness in feedlot cattle vaccination against *Mannheimia haemolytica, Pasteurella multocida*, or *Histophilus somni*.

Overview of Meta-Analysis of Monensin in Dairy Cattle **107**

Todd F. Duffield, Ahmad Rabiee, and Ian J. Lean

Monensin is an ionophore widely used in the dairy cattle industry throughout the world. A large volume of clinical trials have been conducted that have explored efficacy for various metabolic, production, and health outcomes. However, the results of the individual studies have in some cases been contradictory and in others inadequately sized to fully address the objectives particularly for health and production. The meta-analysis of monensin dairy data illustrates an example of the power of this tool for helping to make evidence-based decisions for health management and production consultants. Its importance and utility will continue to grow in future years.

Evidence-Based Early Clinical Detection of Emerging Diseases in Food Animals and Zoonoses: Two Cases **121**

Claude Saegerman, Marie-France Humblet, Sarah Rebecca Porter, Gina Zanella, and Ludovic Martinelle

If diseases of food-producing animals or zoonoses (re-)emerge, early clinical decision making is of major importance. In this particular condition, it is difficult to apply a classic evidence-based veterinary medicine process, because of a lack of available published data. A method based on the partition of field clinical observations (evidences) could be developed as an interesting alternative approach. The classification and regression tree (CART) analysis was used to improve the early clinical detection in two cases of emerging diseases: bovine spongiform encephalopathy (mad cow disease) and bluetongue due to the serotype 8-virus in cattle.

Evidence-Based Practice? An Evolution Is Necessary for Bovine Practitioners, Teachers, and Researchers **133**

Jean-Michel Vandeweerd, Pascal Gustin, and Sébastien Buczinski

We suggest a definition of evidence-based veterinary medicine that takes into account its objectives and practicality. We view it as an information tool that does not replace experience but helps to improve background knowledge and solve clinical foreground questions. It could be defined as the use of accurate, informative, and clear summarized information (abstracts) of high-level research studies that is obtained quickly via free-access databases available via the Internet and that is provided by a proactive veterinary scientific community in search of transparency, accountability, and evidence.

Index **141**

FORTHCOMING ISSUES

July 2012

Mastitis
Pamela L. Ruegg, DVM, MPVM,
Guest Editor

November 2012

Diagnostic Pathology
Vicki Cooper, DVM, PhD,
Guest Editor

RECENT ISSUES

November 2011

Johne's Disease
Michael T. Collins, DVM, PhD,
Guest Editor

July 2011

Ruminant Toxicology
Gary D. Osweiler, DVM, MS, PhD,
Guest Editor

March 2011

Therapeutics and Control of Sheep and Goat Diseases
George C. Fthenakis, DVM, MSc, PhD, and Paula I. Menzies, DVM, MPVM,
Guest Editors

RELATED INTEREST

Veterinary Clinics of North America: Equine Practice
December 2011 (Vol. 27, No. 3)
Clinical Neurology
Thomas J. Divers, DVM, and Amy L. Johnson, DVM, *Guest Editors*

Preface
Evidence-Based Veterinary Medicine

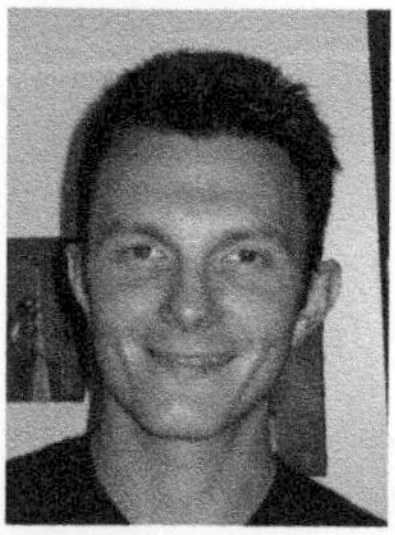
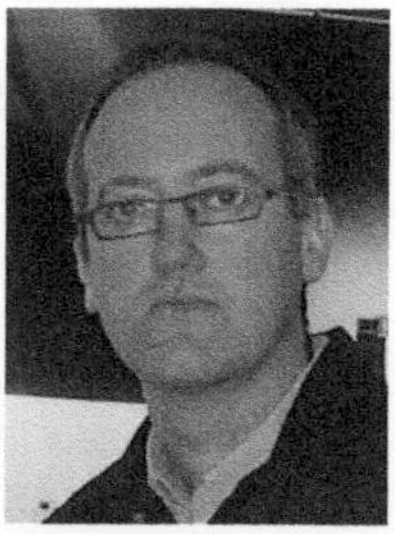

Sébastien Buczinski, Dr Vét, DÉS, MSc Jean-Michel Vandeweerd, DMV, MS
Guest Editors

FROM THE PUBLISHED SCIENTIFIC EVIDENCE TO THE CLINIC . . .

The concept of evidence-based veterinary medicine (EBVM) should be the ultimate goal of every food animal veterinary practitioner or animal scientist. Day after day in our practice, we try to make the best decisions when we treat an animal for a disease, when we suggest a processing protocol for a feedlot producer, or when we choose an estrus synchronization program for a dairy farm. However, despite the fact that we make multiple decisions every day, very few of them are evidence-based. We can suggest to the local dairy producer to treat a cow with a displaced abomasum surgery for the next 3 days with antibiotics, but why not 0, 1, or 2 days? With this example, we understand easily that many of our daily decisions come from our own clinical experience as well as from that of other colleagues, sometimes collected in textbooks. However, EBVM is not only reading published studies. Publication does not imply that the scientific information is of high quality and that it can be extrapolated to the daily veterinary practice. EBVM is also a question of assessing the level of evidence and its applicability to the case.

The practice of EBVM should improve our decision process via a thorough assessment of the available information. To practice EBVM, we must start from a concise practical question we want to answer: for example, for a specific disease, is treatment A better than B? Since we work in food animals, we must focus our search not only on health outcome but also on cost/effectiveness outcome. If treatment A decreases mortality from 0.1% but costs 10 times more, it won't be used on the field. The other steps involve searching the scientific publications that are available to answer the question, assessing their quality, and deciding whether they can be applied to the case. Unfortunately, those different steps may be time consuming. Since busy bovine practitioners may lack time to review all the evidence on every

Vet Clin Food Anim 28 (2012) xiii–xiv
doi:10.1016/j.cvfa.2012.01.003

topic, we truly think that researchers and academics need to present evidence in the form of summarized information that is made available to bovine practitioners.

Systematic reviews of studies are a key component of the EBVM practice. They constitute the highest level of evidence as they are a very critical summary of studies published about a specific topic.

The aim of this special issue is therefore to illustrate how the EBVM approach can be applied to answer practical clinical questions using systematic reviews. After presenting the context of decision-making in the veterinary profession, we describe the concept and method of systematic review. Then, this methodology is used to answer several clinical questions. Strengths and weaknesses are illustrated. We conclude with our own vision of EBVM for the next decade: an information tool that does not replace experience but helps to improve background knowledge and solve clinical foreground questions. EBVM could be defined as the use of accurate, informative, and clear summarized information of high-level research studies that is provided by a proactive veterinary scientific community in search of transparency, accountability, and evidence.

We sincerely want to thank Dr Bob Smith and Mr John Vassallo for allowing us to propose a highly original issue of the *Veterinary Clinics of North America: Food Animal Practice*. We also sincerely want to thank all the contributors of this special issue on EBVM. We know the extra work that was requested with this type of article (systematic reviews). We are convinced that the readers of the *Veterinary Clinics of North America: Food Animal Practice* will appreciate the high quality of this issue that illustrates how EBVM may help decision-making on various topics on beef or dairy medicine.

Sébastien Buczinski, Dr Vét, DÉS, MSc
Département des Sciences Cliniques
Faculté de Médecine Vétérinaire
St-Hyacinthe, Université de Montréal
CP 5000, J2S 7C6 Québec, Canada

Jean-Michel Vandeweerd, DMV, MS
Integrated Veterinary Research Unit - Namur
Research Institute for Life Sciences
Department of Veterinary Medicine
Faculty of Sciences
University of Namur
Rue de Bruxelles 61, 5000 Namur, Belgium

E-mail addresses:
s.buczinski@umontreal.ca (S. Buczinski)
jean-michel.vandeweerd@ulg.ac.be (J.-M. Vandeweerd)

How Can Veterinarians Base Their Medical Decisions on the Best Available Scientific Evidence?

Jean-Michel Vandeweerd, DMV, MS[a,*], Peter Clegg, VetMB, MA, PhD[b], Sébastien Buczinski, Dr Vét, DÉS, MSc[c]

KEYWORDS

- Decision making • Evidence-based medicine
- Scientific evidence • Academic research • Education

Today veterinarians play an important role in 5 related fields of work: public health, biomedical research, global food safety and security, ecosystem health, as well as in the more traditional role of caring for animals.[1] As a consequence of both societal needs and expectations of the profession, external demands on the profession are increasingly critical and far-reaching. It is necessary for the veterinary community to both demonstrate the validity and robustness of their decisions, as well as providing accountability. Mistakes in management of specific disease events can jeopardize the biosecurity of an entire region, several countries, or even the whole world.[2] Veterinarians involved in food production are required, not only to identify what is the best therapeutic option for farm animals but also what is the most cost-effective and economic approach. At the level of the individual animal, much of the time of a veterinary practitioner, as in human medicine, is spent in making diagnostic, therapeutic, and preventive decisions in a complex and uncertain environment.[3,4]

The veterinary profession has ethical obligation to provide effective and safe actions in a market that changes with more price-conscious clients and a more

[a] Integrated Veterinary Research Unit - Namur Research Institute for Life Sciences, Department of Veterinary Medicine, Faculty of Sciences, University of Namur, Rue de Bruxelles 61, 5000 Namur, Belgium
[b] Department of Veterinary Clinical Science and Husbandry, University of Liverpool, Leahurst, Neston, Cheshire, United Kingdom
[c] Département des Sciences Cliniques, Faculté de Médecine Vétérinaire, St-Hyacinthe, Université de Montréal, CP 5000, J2S 7C6 Québec, Canada
* Corresponding author. Rue verte 208, 4040 Herstal, Belgium.
E-mail address: jean-michel.vandeweerd@ulg.ac.be

Vet Clin Food Anim 28 (2012) 1–11
doi:10.1016/j.cvfa.2011.12.001 vetfood.theclinics.com
0749-0720/12/$ – see front matter

demanding regulatory environment.[5] Careful and increasingly evidence-based decisions are required to minimize the liability risks.[6] For veterinarians to be successful over the broad and complex range of services and activities in which they operate, they must possess an extensive knowledge base and acquire the skills that will ensure their continuing success and excellence in making appropriate decisions in all their requisite specialities.[2]

In human medicine, several tools have been designed to support medical decision such as decision analysis, decision tables, and decision trees. The evidence-based medicine (EBM) approach defined by Sackett and colleagues is another one.[7] EBM refers to the conscientious, explicit, and judicious use of current best evidence from research for the care of an individual patient.

The concept of EBM was first described in human medicine in the early 1990s and was introduced to veterinary medicine in the early 2000s. Since 2003, several initiatives have been taken to develop the practice of EBM in the veterinary field, largely using the concepts and tools of human medicine. However, 10 years later, it is not clear that the EBM approach promulgated in human medicine can be applied to the same extent to veterinary medicine and in the same way. EBM has the potential to help veterinarians to make more informed decisions, but obstacles to its widespread adoption have been described.[8] It is therefore essential to determine what hinders the adoption and practice of EBM. In particular we need to better understand the process of decision making in veterinary practice and to explore perception of EBM by practitioners.

We postulate that an evidence-based veterinary medicine (EBVM) is mandatory, that the way it is practiced in human medicine is currently inadequate for veterinary practice, and that appropriate tools of scientific information must be designed and developed.

PRINCIPLES OF EBM

To practice EBM, some skills are necessary. Several textbooks that summarize the process in an easily accessible manner are now available, written specifically for both medicine[9] and veterinary medicine.[10,11] Although it is possible to understand and practice the principles of EBM without advanced knowledge of clinical epidemiology, this discipline is the core of EBM; this may be an advantage for bovine practitioners who used applied epidemiology during preventive medicine in dairy or beef herds.

Classically, the EBM approach is composed of 5 steps[8]:

1. The first step is to translate the problem into an answerable question. A technique has been advocated based on the so-called PICO and PECOT principles. These acronyms remind the clinician of the different parts of a well-formulated question. "P" is for "patient" or "problem." "I" (or "E") is for "intervention" (or "exposures"). The intervention could be a diagnosis, therapeutic intervention, prognostic factor or exposure. "C" is for the "control" group. It defines the alternative; it may be one treatment versus either another treatment or no treatment. It is sometimes useful to consider "doing nothing" as an alternative. "O" is for clinical "outcome," which is what the clinician hopes to accomplish, measure, improve, or effect by their intervention or treatment. The "time" frame ("T") during which the outcome is expected to occur is sometimes included in the question. Although this technique may appear to be awkward, clinicians who use the PICO and PECOT systems are able to identify concepts and descriptors (keywords) that allow literature databases to be searched more effectively for quality articles.[12,13] An example of a well-formulated question would be relating

to a cow with mastitis due to *Staphylococcus aureus* infection (P); specifically questioning whether intramammary treatments (I) are better than systemic treatments (C) in both treating the condition and improving the production (O).

2. The second step is to search the literature to identify a list of publications that are related to the clinical question. This requires the use of databases accessed via the Internet or institutional intranets. Databases frequently used include MEDLINE (via PubMed and available on http://www.ncbi.nlm.nih.gov/pubmed/), Agricola for food animal topics hosted by the US Department of Agriculture, and Commonwealth Agricultural Bureau (CAB) abstracts. The availability of CAB is largely limited to academic institutions, while PubMed is freely accessible. To elaborate the query, descriptors (keywords) must be identified. PubMed has its own list of descriptors but the keywords in the question designed in Step 1 may not be suitable. For example, should we use "cow" or "cattle"? Spelling of conditions may also vary between different forms of a language, for instance, "haemorrhage/hemorrhage." Therefore, it is advised to use the MeSH Database (MEDLINE SubHeadings). In PubMed, a demonstration of its use is available at http://www.ncbi.nlm.nih.gov/mesh?itool=sidebar. Descriptors are then integrated in a query that combines the keywords with Boolean operators (AND, OR, NOT). However, PubMed does not always provide adequate indexing and abstracting to all literature relevant to veterinary clinical questions, and it may be useful to perform a free search.[14] This is the introduction of words in the query field without using the MeSH Database and Boolean operators. An example of query to identify publications concerning the usefulness of anti-inflammatory drugs in feedlot calves with bovine respiratory disease (BRD) would be: ("non steroidal anti-inflammatory" OR "flunixin" OR "ketoprofen" or "tolfenamic acid" OR "meloxicam" OR "aspirin") AND ("respiratory disease" OR "pneumonia" or "lung disease") AND ("bovine" OR "cattle" OR "calves" OR "ox" OR "steer" OR "heifer").
3. The third step consists of critical appraisal of external evidence that enlightens the clinical question. It is here that the work of EBM is largely accomplished, through assessment of internal validity and quality of publications that were identified in the database searches. An initial selection can be accomplished on the basis of the date of publication. As authors are supposed to review the literature to write their article, most recent articles should summarize the content of less recent publications. Then selection can be refined on the basis of 2 principles.

   - First, the levels of evidence can be summarized in a pyramid designed to help the clinician to order the commonly applied study designs (**Fig. 1**).[15] Studies toward the top of the pyramid provide "stronger" evidence because the design of these studies limits possible biases (systematic error) and adequate statistical analysis is performed, (thus limiting random error). Yusuf and colleagues further categorized the levels of evidence.[16] Class A evidence is the "best" and is derived from randomized, double-blind, placebo-controlled clinical trials. Class B evidence is derived from high-quality clinical trials using historical controls, and Class C evidence is from uncontrolled case series. The least reliable is Class D evidence, which is derived from anecdotal clinical reports or expert opinion. The top level of evidence consists of meta-analyses of randomized controlled trials (RCTs) (ie, a process of synthesizing research results by using various statistical methods to retrieve, select, and combine results from previous separate but related RCTs). Recognizing and understanding study designs are helped considerably by having a basic knowledge of clinical epidemiology.

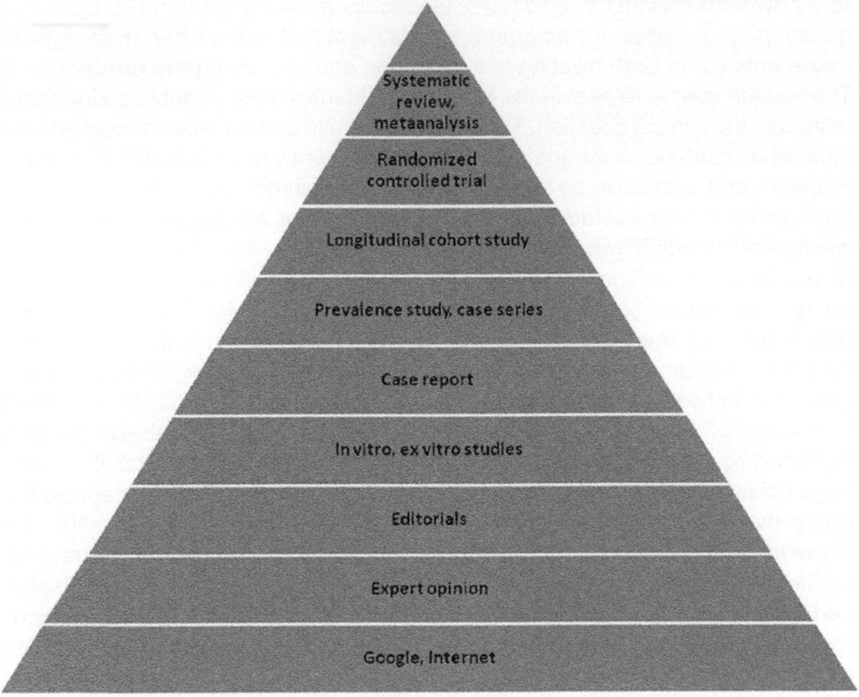

Fig. 1. Pyramid of evidence: designs at the top of the pyramid carry a higher level of evidence.

- Second, some study designs are more suitable to answer a specific type of clinical question (**Table 1**). For example, RCTs are ideal to provide information relating to the efficacy of a therapeutic intervention.
- This initial selection is often performed only through reading information provided in titles and abstracts of an article. Frequently busy practitioners may rely on this information alone, although it is always sensible accessing the full article and critically appraise its entire content.
- **Table 2** displays a list of publications identified with PubMed referring to the treatment of bovine interdigital dermatitis. Publications have been selected to show the variety of study designs.

4. In the fourth step, the critical appraisal process alone is normally insufficient to arrive at the best clinical decision for the patient. The final therapeutic approach should

Table 1
Some study designs are more adequate to answer some clinical questions

Question	Study Design
Treatment	Randomized controlled trial
Risk	Retrospective cohort study, case-control study
Frequency	Cross-sectional study (prevalence study)
Diagnostic	Cross-sectional study
Prognosis	Prospective cohort study

Table 2
Possible study designs are listed in the right column

Reference	Possible Study Designs
1. Green et al. Public understanding of food risks in four European countries: a qualitative study. Eur J Public Health 2005;15:523–7. 2. Hernandez et al. Comparison of topical application of oxytetracycline and four nonantibiotic solutions for treatment of papillomatous digital dermatitis in dairy cows. J Am Vet Med Assoc 1999;214:688–90. 3. Moore et al. Efficacy of a nonantimicrobial cream administered topically for treatment of digital dermatitis in dairy cattle. J Am Vet Med Assoc 2001;219:1435–8. 4. Lischer et al. Effect of therapeutic dietary biotin on the healing of uncomplicated sole ulcers in dairy cattle—a double blinded controlled study. Vet J 2002;163:51–60. 5. Zeiner et al. Effect of different claw trimming methods on the pressure distribution under the bovine claw—an in vitro study. Berl Munch Tierarztl Wochenschr 2007;120:165–72. 6. Trostle et al. Use of antimicrobial-impregnated polymethyl methacrylate beads for treatment of chronic, refractory septic arthritis and osteomyelitis of the digit in a bull. J Am Vet Med Assoc 1996;208:404–7. 7. Kasari et al. Use of autogenous cancellous bone graft for treatment of osteolytic defects in the phalanges of three cattle. J Am Vet Med Assoc 1992;201:1053–7. 8. Desrochers et al. Use of facilitated ankylosis in the treatment of septic arthritis of the distal interphalangeal joint in cattle: 12 cases (1987-1992). J Am Vet Med Assoc 1995;206:1923–7. 9. Holzhauer et al. Herd and cow-level prevalence of sole ulcers in The Netherlands and associated-risk factors. Prev Vet Med 2008;85:125–35. 10. Hernandez et al. Comparison of milk yield in dairy cows with different degrees of lameness. J Am Vet Med Assoc 2005;227:1292–6. 11. Bicalho et al. Strategies to analyze milk losses caused by diseases with potential incidence throughout the lactation: a lameness example. J Dairy Sci 2008;91:2653–61.	Experimentation • Clinical trial ○ Without control ○ Controlled [2] ▪ Randomized [3] ▪ Double blind [4] ▪ Cross-over ▪ Historical control • Ex vivo/in vitro study [5] Observation • Qualitative study [1] • Quantitative study ○ Descriptive ▪ Single case report [6] ▪ Case report [7] ▪ Case series [8] ▪ Cross-sectional study [9] ▪ Ecological study ○ Analytic ▪ Longitudinal study • Prospective cohort [10] • Retrospective cohort [11] • Case-control [11]

Numbers in brackets refer to the examples given in the left column.

integrate the best scientific information with clinical expertise and an understanding of the unique features of individual patients (and clients). The context must be taken into account. The relevance and agreement of the identified publications with other articles relating to the same subject must also be determined. This step refers to the external validity of the publications. For example, a report describing therapeutic options of BRD in small dairy farms in the Swiss Alps may not be relevant for a practitioner dealing with North American feedlots.

5. The fifth step is continuous self-assessment of the decision-making process and outcomes, so as to improve future appraisals.

HISTORY AND OBSTACLES

The term "evidence-based medicine" first appeared in the veterinary literature in about 2000 to counteract emerging alternative veterinary therapies, with the argument that these could not be validated by high quality scientific information.[8] Other initiatives in favor of EBM became prominent in 2003, for instance in the field of canine medicine with an exemplar review by Olivry and colleagues that identified the best evidence relating to the pharmacotherapy of canine atopy.[17] In equine practice, the concept of EBM was gaining prominence. Peter Rossdale edited a special issue of the *Equine Veterinary Journal* to promote EBM and announced that the journal would introduce a specific section devoted to articles specifically meeting the criteria of EBM.[18] In the same issue, Rossdale presented what he called "the guide for those who wish to enter the subject of Evidence Based Veterinary Medicine": the book published by Cockcroft and Holmes.[10]

After 2003, a number of general articles about EBVM have been published. These cover topics such as searching the literature, critical reviews, statistics and power, study design, allocation concealment and randomization, statistical methods, the Consolidated Standards of Reporting Trials (CONSORT) statement, and reporting observational studies. The key concepts of EBM have been developed in different veterinary disciplines and have also been promoted in the German, Dutch, and French languages.[8] In 2007, 2 special issues about EBM were published in *Veterinary Clinics of North America* in equine and small animal medicine, largely describing the human approach and attempting to apply the principles of this approach to small animal and equine practice.[19,20] This approach can also be used in cattle introducing a dimension referring to cost-effectiveness of the intervention that will have a big impact on the application of the new treatment or preventive option in the field.

With this growing number of evidence-based resources being developed for use in veterinary medicine, academicians, practitioners, specialists, and students were encouraged to embrace the positive elements of EBM. However, several obstacles to its widespread adoption have been reported.[8] They include (1) the lack of high-quality patient-centered research such as RCTs, (2) the absence of adequate searching techniques and accessibility to scientific data bases, (3) the limited number of open access journals, (4) the need for basic understanding of clinical epidemiology by veterinarians, and (5) the inadequacy of EBM tools to the busy daily practice due to the limited time available to bovine veterinarians to keep up to date with the large quantity of scientific literature.

Considering those issues, we suggest that perception of EBM should be investigated at a larger scale, in order to build the most useful and adequate tools for veterinary practitioners.[21]

PERCEPTION OF EBM

The results of a qualitative study in Europe demonstrated that the EBM approach is not frequently applied by veterinarians to better inform their decisions (J.M. Vandeweerd and colleagues, personal communication, 2011). These findings were similar to those of McKenzie and colleagues in a survey of practicing veterinarians in the United States relating to their familiarity with the terms and concepts of EBM and their attitudes toward it.[21] In Mc Kenzie's study, 5000 veterinarians were invited to participate via a printed letter, and 119 web-based questionnaires were completed (response rate of about 2.5%). Between 25.2% and 76.5% responded that they were not familiar with common EBVM-related terms. Respondents clearly relied on research summaries, consensus statements, and protocols promulgated by professional organizations to a much greater extent than on the use of independent peer-reviewed literature.[21]

These findings highlight the needs to train veterinarians to accurately identify and evaluate scientific information and to develop tools to optimize the time spent in query and assessment of publications. EBM is rarely used by practitioners, and there is a risk that if EBM tools are not adapted to specific types of practice, such as food animal medicine, the situation will not improve. This analysis of obstacles and perception has important implications on education, research strategy, and publication of scientific findings.

EDUCATION

At the patient/population level, qualitative studies relating to veterinary medicine suggest that decision-making proceeds also on the recognition-primed decision-making model, as in human medicine (J.M. Vandeweerd and colleagues, personal communication, 2011).[4] Veterinarians recognize that a clinical situation fits a particular pattern, and based on this, make management decisions. They are often not conscious of making decisions but act in response to the pattern of the situation in front of them. A quick decision is made based on what appears to be the most suitable solution by comparing the actual situation (case) to what they have experienced in the past. Even when a veterinarian has no experience of a similar situation, there is often need for a rapid decision. This is not perceived as an issue as veterinarians are normally aware about the follow-up of the case, and any eventual outcome, and will reassess the initial option as required. Interestingly, when the situation is complex or encountered for the first time, veterinarians may not apply a systematic hypothetico-deductive approach but use more or less an "attempt and mistake" process to validate or reject a list of decision options that has been built from their own experience, the experience of colleagues or other professionals, and information gained from the Internet and other sources.

If we accept the idea of knowledge explosion and that nobody can master all the knowledge about all animals, this model has several implications on the way education of veterinarians should be organized.

The first one is the necessity to clearly and accurately identify the quantity and nature of knowledge to teach. It should be the necessary background to understand the content of abstracts, publications, or other sources of information. In other words, it is important to identify what students should be taught, so in the future they can learn quickly what they do not know.

The second one refers to the necessity to develop the skills to identify and evaluate scientific information. This means that undergraduates should be trained in clinical epidemiology and EBM.

The third aspect to consider relates to the necessity to train undergraduates in the management of doubt and mistake, the scientific and informed decision may be understood as the revision of a less scientific and less informed initial decision. Therefore, students should be able to answer to questions such as, "If you have made a quick decision, what do you do now to confirm or infirm this decision, to make another or better one, to explain it to the owner?" Training sessions should give the possibility to students to understand several steps of decision-making: (1) take immediate decisions whose effects are not irreversible and which are cost effective; (2) assess initial decisions and identify weakest points; (3) obtain colleague or expert opinion, and identify relevant scientific information, that may modify the plan of action; and (4) explain and justify revision of the diagnostic or therapeutic plan to the client, which is sometimes perceived as confessing a mistake, an excessive risk, a loss of time or a wastage of resource. This does not mean that the rationale decision-making model should not be taught to students.[4] It is certainly useful to make the decisional process more explicit, but it is also essential to conceptualize a more realistic decision model, inspired from the process reported and practiced by veterinarians.

Lifelong education in EBM is also an essential requirement and an effort needs to be made to include the discipline in the undergraduate veterinary curriculum. This discipline should also be taught to experienced practitioners via continuing professional development and targeted publications. It is also important that speakers in veterinary congress agree to briefly expose how the information they present was assessed, to provide its level of evidence, and give how the practitioner could use the information practically. For food animal veterinarians, economic-based decision is also of primary importance, since not only the medical efficacy of a treatment but also the cost-effectiveness influence decision. The cost-benefit analysis has a huge impact on the profitability of a farm. Using a brief example: if a treatment for BRD results in a 10% decrease of mortality in North American feedlot but costs twice the price of the actual therapeutic plan in a feedlot with an actual 30% of BRD morbidity and 2% of BRD mortality, the veterinarian would not be perceived as a professional in convincing his (her) client to change his strategy facing to BRD. In doing so, the expenses would be greater than the benefits and therefore would lead a reduced profit for the farmer. Undergraduates should therefore be trained to economics and management strategies.

At a more global level, the concept of One World of Veterinary Medicine implies that veterinarians become better connected to the world around to play their full societal role and gain new public recognition and esteem.[1] Enforcing the search and the application of the best evidence must be part of the educational transformation that veterinary schools must lead to reaffirm the social contract of veterinarians.

RESEARCH STRATEGY AND PUBLICATION

Good evidence is based on well-designed and rigorous research and must be available and useful to practitioners and policy makers.[8] Several strategies could be developed to counteract the obstacles to strong methodology.

- Recruiting clinical material from primary first opinion practice has been proposed to improve the sample size and statistical power of studies.[22] Computerized data mining systems could also be developed to collect data in the field and facilitate participation of practitioners in research.[23] This may be difficult in practice due to the absence of sufficient funds to allow this type of data management.
- The RCTs generally require considerable resources and are often beyond the range of many veterinary researchers.[24] As a consequence, retrospective observational studies (such as longitudinal/cohort studies and case-control studies) are prevalent in the veterinary literature. It might be better to aim to conduct a good retrospective study rather than attempt a difficult RCT that ends up being poorly conducted.[24,25] The results in terms of strength of evidence are likely to be greater for the former than for the latter.
- Instruments for validating outcomes are not always available and their development should be encouraged to provide a standardized means for clinical assessment of the efficacy of veterinary treatments.[26] A good example of this

lack of standardization are clinical scores. In using the example of BRD treatment, we can easily compare different interventions in 3 different RCTs in term of rectal temperature 24 hours after treatments or BRD mortality rate. However, it would be very difficult to compare clinical score since in one study the depression score would have more weight that in the other, or would be absent in the clinical score presented in a third article. Accurately defining accurate outcomes measurement is a key feature to be able to compare different articles on the same topic.
- It is also important to ensure that research is critically evaluated in terms of transparency, completeness, and accuracy, and there has been progress recently in the development of reporting guidelines for veterinary research.[27,28]

Other authors have suggested that, as in human medicine, information such as systematic reviews and CATs (critically appraised topics) should be available so that practitioners devote their scarce reading time to selected quality scientific information.[29,30] Systematic reviews are currently rare in veterinary medicine and their format has not been completely standardized as in human medicine.[31] Though systematic reviews may give the impression of a strong criticism by scientists on the work of their colleagues, transparency and accountability policies are widely accepted strategies to drive quality improvement and stimulate consumer choice. It is therefore important to work on the availability of such informational tools for the use of practitioners. It is also essential to have sight of more clinical studies. In particular, less confidentiality and more open access to data relating to medicinal products or feed additives are required to better inform veterinary surgeons. In addition, guidelines should be elaborated to reach a standardization of systematic review of trials and observational studies to limit heterogeneity of results and ensure fair comparisons between studies. Transparency is also one of the main objectives of the World Organisation for Animal Health (OIE) to ensure knowledge of the world animal health situation.[2]

SUMMARY

With the advent of a One World-One Health concept, veterinarians will play a central role, at the level of trading zones (such as the European Union), countries, food production farms, and individual animals. They will be mandated to produce, interpret, communicate, and apply scientific information in the best possible way to make informed decisions and take adequate actions. The principles of EBM will help the accomplishment of this mission. However, for the moment, we may still have the impression of two separate worlds, the academic research on one side and the reality of practice on the other side. There is a need to join them, perhaps by making efforts to include the huge amount of clinical data from practice into research. Both worlds should also meet in the field of education where students should be trained in the complexity and reality of decision making. Adequate information tools should be developed to take into account the preoccupations and obstacles to practitioners working in the field.

REFERENCES

1. King LJ. One world of veterinary medicine. Rev Sci Tech 2009;28:463–80.
2. Ben Jebara K. The OIE World Animal Health Information System: the role of OIE Reference Laboratories and Collaborating Centres in disease reporting. Rev Sci Tech 2010;29:451–8.

3. Cockcroft PD, Holmes MA. Decision analysis, models and economics as evidence. In: Handbook of evidence-based veterinary medicine. Oxford (UK): Blackwell Publishing; 2003. p. 154–81.
4. Del Mar C, Doust J, Glasziou P. Clinical thinking: evidence, communication and decision making. Oxford (UK): Blackwell Publishing; 2006.
5. Vos JH, Deleu SA, Heling W, et al. Veterinarians: 'watch your affairs!' Tijdschr Diergeneeskd 2000;125:542–51.
6. O'Connell D, Bonvicini KA. Addressing disappointment in veterinary practice. Vet Clin North Am Small Anim Pract 2007;37:135–49.
7. Sackett DL, Rosenberg WM, Gray JA, et al. Evidence based medicine: what it is and what it isn't. BMJ 1996;312:71–2.
8. Vandeweerd JM, Kirschvink N, Clegg P, et al. Is evidence-based medicine so evident in veterinary research and practice? History, obstacles and perspectives. Vet J 2011. [Epub ahead of print].
9. Greenhalgh T. How to read a paper. The basics of evidence based medicine, 2nd ed. London: BMJ Books; 2001.
10. Cockcroft P, Holmes M. Handbook of evidence-based veterinary medicine. Oxford (UK): Blackwell Publishing; 2003.
11. Vandeweerd JM, Saegerman C. Guide pratique de médecine factuelle vétérinaire. Paris: Les Editions du Point Vétérinaire; 2009.
12. Cabell CH, Schardt C, Sanders L, et al. Resident utilization of information technology. J Gen Intern Med 2001;16:838–44.
13. Villaneuva EV, Burrows EA, Fennessy PA. Improving question formulation for use in appraisal in a tertiary care setting: a randomized controlled trial. BMC Med Informed Decis Making 2001;1:4.
14. Murphy SA. Searching for veterinary evidence: strategies and resources for locating clinical research. Vet Clin North Am Small Anim Pract 2007;37:433–45.
15. Sackett DL, Straus SE, Richardson WS, et al. Evidence-based medicine. How to practice and teach EBM. New York: Churchill Livingstone; 1997.
16. Yusuf S, Cairns JA, Camm AJ, et al. Evidence-based cardiology. London: BMJ Publishing Group; 1998.
17. Olivry T, Mueller RS, and the International Task Force on Canine Atopic Dermatitis. Evidence-based veterinary dermatology: a systematic review of the pharmacotherapy of canine atopic dermatitis. Vet Dermatol 2003;14:121–46.
18. Rossdale P. Objectivity versus subjectivity in medical progress. Equine Vet J 2003; 35:331–2.
19. Schmidt PL. Evidence-based veterinary medicine: evolution, revolution, or repackaging of veterinary practice? Vet Clin North Am Small Anim Pract 2007;37(3):409–17.
20. Williamson KK, Davis MS. Evidence-based respiratory medicine in horses. Vet Clin North Am Equine Pract 2007;23(2):215–27.
21. McKenzie B. Practitioner survey: Evidence-Based Veterinary Medicine Association. 2011. Available at: http://ebvma.org.
22. Mair TS, Cohen ND. AEEP and BEVA member-based observational research studies: a novel approach to epidemiological and evidence-based medicine studies in equine medicine. Equine Vet J 2003;35:339–40.
23. Vandeweerd JM., Davies J, Desbrosse F. A data management system to tackle the challenges of equine practice at the beginning of the XXI century. In: Proceedings of SIVE Congress. Bologna, Italy, 2006, p. 150–1.
24. Parkin T. Evidence based medicine: an academic's viewpoint—not so different to that of the clinician. J Small Anim Pract 2010;51:509–10.

25. Dohoo IR, Leslie K, DesCôteaux L, et al. A meta-analysis review of the effects of recombinant bovine somatotropin. 1. Methodology and effects on production. Can J Vet Res 2003;67:241–51.
26. Schulz KS. The Outcomes Measures Program: what's in it for you? Vet Surg 2007;36:715–6.
27. More SJ. Improving the quality of reporting in veterinary journals: how far do we need to go with reporting guidelines? Vet J 2010;184:249–50.
28. O'Connor AM, Sargeant JM, Gardner IA, et al. The REFLECT statement: methods and processes of creating reporting guidelines for randomized controlled trials for livestock and food safety. Prev Vet Med 2010;93:11–8.
29. Marr CM, Newton JR. Clinical evidence articles in Equine Veterinary Journal: progress since inception. Equine Vet J 2006;38:110–2.
30. Holmes MA. Philosophical foundations of evidence-based medicine for veterinary clinicians. J Am Vet Med Assoc 2009;235:1035–9.
31. Glasziou P, Irwig L, Bain C, et al. Systematic reviews in health care. Cambridge (UK): Cambridge University Press; 2001.

Using Systematic Reviews to Critically Appraise the Scientific Information for the Bovine Veterinarian

Jean-Michel Vandeweerd, DMV, MS[a,*], Peter Clegg, VetMB, MA, PhD[b],
V. Hougardy, BSc[c], Sébastien Buczinski, Dr Vét, DÉS, MSc[d]

KEYWORDS

• Bovine • Systematic reviews • Scientific evidence
• Evidence-based medicine

As in human medicine, information tools such as systematic reviews and CATs (critically appraised topics) should be available to busy veterinary practitioners so that they devote their scarce reading time to selected quality and summarized scientific information.[1,2] According to the principles of evidence-based medicine (EBM), systematic reviews are the more appropriate way to summarize the information that is available to answer a clinical question or a herd health issue. Such reviews aim to evaluate and interpret all available evidence relevant to a particular question.[3] Using this approach, a concerted attempt is made to identify all relevant primary research, a standardized appraisal of quality is made, and then studies of acceptable quality are systematically synthesized. The term "systematic" refers to this process. This differs from a traditional review in which previous work is described but neither systematically identified nor assessed for quality. This systematic approach is particularly important in order to avoid bias due to the personal perspective of the authors performing the review. A systematic review needs to be conducted as a scientific original analytic article with a complete material and methods section indicating to the reader how the information was assessed in order to be repeatable. The term

The authors have nothing to disclose.

[a] Integrated Veterinary Research Unit - Namur Research Institute for Life Sciences, Department of Veterinary Medicine, Faculty of Sciences, University of Namur, Rue de Bruxelles 61, 5000 Namur, Belgium
[b] Department of Veterinary Clinical Science and Husbandry, University of Liverpool, Leahurst, Neston, Cheshire, UK
[c] CHR–Site de La Citadelle, University of Liège, Liège, Belgium
[d] Département des Sciences Cliniques, Faculté de Médecine Vétérinaire, St-Hyacinthe, Université de Montréal, CP 5000, J2S 7C6 Québec, Canada
* Corresponding author.
E-mail address: jean-michel.vandeweerd@fundp.ac.be

Vet Clin Food Anim 28 (2012) 13–21
doi:10.1016/j.cvfa.2011.12.002 vetfood.theclinics.com
0749-0720/12/$ – see front matter

"meta-analysis" is used when a systematic review consists of a quantitative process of synthesizing research results by using various statistical methods to retrieve, select, and combine results from previous independent but related studies. A meta-analysis can be only performed when studies available are comparable in terms of population, definition of treatments, and outcome measurements.[4]

The aim of this article is to explain what systematic reviews are and to suggest a methodology of conducting and reporting them that would improve transparency for both scientists and veterinary practitioners interested in ruminant health issues. Different aspect of the methods will be illustrated in subsequent articles in the present issue of the *Veterinary Clinics of North America: Food Animal Practice.*

MATERIAL AND METHODS OF A SYSTEMATIC REVIEW

A systematic review generally requires considerably more effort than a traditional review.[3] It involves a number of discrete steps. The method is also influenced by the type of question that is asked. It may concern (1) the etiology or risk factors of a disease; (2), the frequency or rate of a condition or disease, (3) the diagnostic accuracy of a sign, symptom or test, (4) the prediction and prognosis of an event, or (5) the treatment or prevention of a disease. Consequently different methods of systematic review may be considered. In this article, we will focus on the material and methods to review clinical trials or experiments.

Literature Search

Finding all relevant information is a difficult task. Ideally, literature should be found among the 22,000 published biomedical journals (it is to note that MEDLINE only indexes 3700 of these) and also in the "grey literature" such as conference proceedings, theses, and unpublished studies. Several strategies may be used to improve the search: (1) using a well-formulated and focused question, (2) breaking down study question into components with Boolean operators, (3) using different databases, (4) using synonyms in the query, (5) using filters of databases that can sort studies by methodologic design, (6) consulting existing reviews and the bibliographies of recent articles on the subject, and (7) writing to experts or colleagues.

One of the key features to perform a systematic review is to formulate a precise and focused answerable question concerning the area of interest of the article. To illustrate this step we can take the following example: "Is systemic antibiotic treatment useful in the healing rate and milk production in cases of acute coliform mastitis in dairy cows?" Using the PICO principle, we can identify several concepts: (P) **P**atient: dairy cows, (I) **I**ntervention: systemic antibiotic treatment, (C) **C**omparison: no systemic antibiotic treatment, and (O) **O**utcome: healing rate and milk production. A clear identification of key words helps make a successful search with databases.

The next step is to convert the clinical question to queries using Boolean operators (AND, OR, NOT). Queries will then be submitted to specific databases. The more commonly used database is MEDLINE since it is free access and can therefore be widely used, in contrast to Ovid, which requires an access fee. Agricola can also be used and is of primary interest for studies performed by US Food and Drug Administration (FDA). Google Scholar is also a database that can be consulted to assess the information available on the clinical question.

It is advised to repeat the search using different synonyms and queries to increase the chance to identify all relevant publications.

If the number of identified information sources is too high, different filters can be used to reduce the amount of references that are obtained (eg, by limiting the list of references to randomized controlled trials [RCTs], or by excluding letters to the editor or case reports). The filter allows the investigators to spare their time by excluding references with a low level of evidence from an EBM perspective. These publications of lower level of evidence should be used in the review only for topics with a low prevalence rate or where publications are scant. For example, it is very unlikely to obtain several randomized controlled trials that could be used to answer to the question: "Does pericardiostomy lead to a better short term outcome than pericardial drainage in adult cows with traumatic pericarditis?"

Next, the authors could consult the bibliographic references of existing reviews and recent textbooks on the topic. However, using such sources, it is often difficult to know whether the list of the bibliographic references is exhaustive and how the authors of the reviews have built their list. Unfortunately, this is frequently the case in bovine medicine as reviews are mainly performed by "experts" who perform an authoritarian (opinion-based) rather than an authoritative (evidence-based) review.

Finally, investigators should try to obtain unpublished trials or data communicated at international congresses that have never been published. In contacting the corresponding authors, they could increase the amount of information available for their systematic review. This method has been mentioned as a valuable tool to assess the level of information.[4]

All articles are obtained and then fully appraised.

Selecting and Excluding Studies

First, it must be clearly stated which studies were eligible (ie, could be assessed for their scientific quality) and which ones were finally selected (ie, were assessed for their scientific quality). The presentation of these data may be facilitated by the use a flow chart diagram with the number of articles initially obtained and of those that were rejected at each step. Articles obtained by methods other than web searches should also be indicated. An example of flow chart is given in **Fig. 1**. The criteria that are used to select or exclude the eligible studies should be clearly stated. Selection and exclusion criteria often refer to the study design (eg, authors could only consider clinical trials and reject observational prospective or retrospective studies) and to the outcome measures (for example, authors could only include studies investigating semi-objective measures like a clinical examination by a veterinarian, and not a subjective measure as the owner's opinion).

Appraising the Quality of Studies

The objective of the "Material and Methods" section is to enable the readers to repeat the study if required. However, in some systematic reviews, the criteria used for the assessment of the methodological quality of trials lack the transparency that is fundamental for evaluation. Some may only describe quality criteria in the most general terms that are not sufficiently informative for any reader.

In human medicine, a number of checklists and guidelines have been published about how to report trials (CONSORT [CONsolidated Standards of Reporting Trials] statement)[5] and observational research (STROBE [Strengthening the Reporting of Observational Studies in Epidemiology]).[6] They can be applied to evaluate the quality of research studies.[7] Recently, guidelines have been published in veterinary medicine.[8,9]

It is out of the scope of this article to review the recommendations for every type of study design. We rather describe an original method that was used recently to review RCTs in veterinary medicine as we think it nicely illustrates the concept of quality assessment in systematic reviews.[10] It also educates the reader about several aspects of clinical epidemiology and, importantly, ensures transparency of the quality

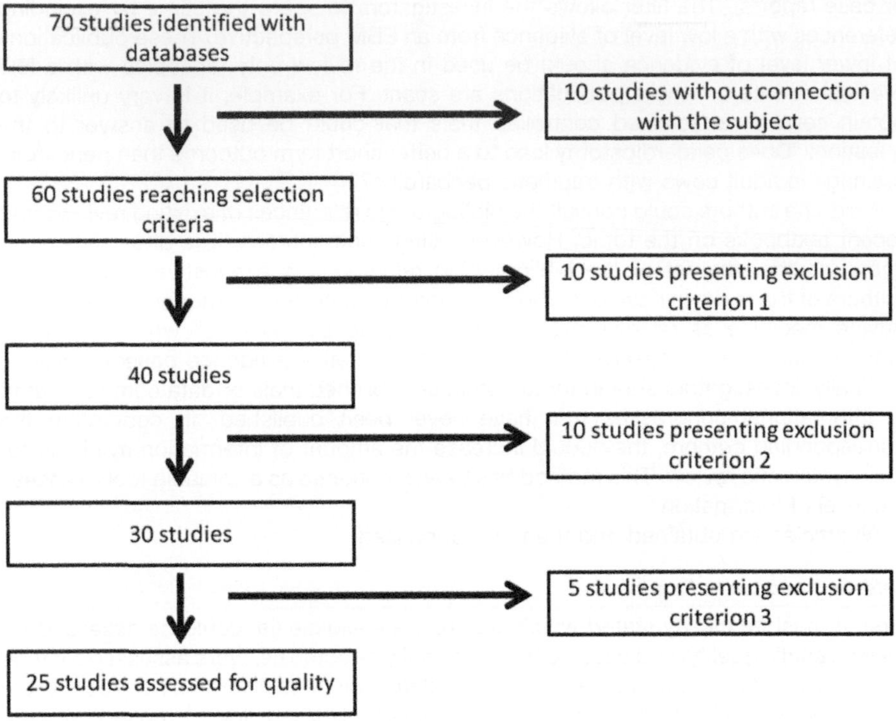

Fig. 1. Example of flow chart describing the selection and exclusion process of studies that were identified with databases.

assessment of studies. This method of evaluation is based on the one proposed by the FDA.[11] It includes an evaluation of internal validity (step 1) and of external validity (steps 2 and 3). The statistically significance of the effect (step 4) and global level of evidence (step 5) are also determined.

For step 1, evaluation criteria are elaborated from several resources: the CONSORT Statement and the recommendations of the Center of Evidence Based Medicine of Oxford (http://www.cebm.net/index.aspx?o=1157). Several question items are listed in a chart (**Box 1**), which is used to evaluate publications. The maximum possible score of quality is 100%. Arbitrarily, studies are of high, intermediate, and low quality, if their scores are higher than 60%, between 45% and 60%, and below 45%, respectively. The scores for the different question items can be reported in **Box 1**. Ideally, at least 2 reviewers should take part in the quality assessment of studies. They should fully discuss any conflicts with each other to resolve any discrepancies.

In step 2, the quantity of published information is evaluated on the basis of the number of studies published and the number of individuals tested. A number of studies can be set arbitrarily and considered adequate by investigators. A sample size can also be set arbitrarily that is considered adequate for each group; this number can be based on power calculation performed in the most representative of the selected studies, if available. This process is usually arbitrary because usually the results are from a low numbers of studies, relating to the same therapeutic intervention with only a low number of individuals within those studies. Globally, quantity is considered adequate

Box 1
Questions used to assess the quality of trials

Title and summary (2/100)

Title and abstract: identification of the study design in the title is present (1%); structured summary of trial design, methods, results, and conclusions is provided (1%)

Introduction (2/100)

Background and objectives: scientific background and explanation of rationale are explained (1%); specific objectives or hypotheses are explained (1%)

Material and methods (48/100)

Trial design: the trial is controlled (1) and allocation ratio is described (1%); reference is made to an ethical protocol (1%)

Participants: eligibility criteria for participants (2%), settings, locations where the data were collected (2%), inclusion criteria (2%), exclusion criteria (2%), are detailed

Interventions: the interventions for each group are described with sufficient details to allow replication (5%) and no additional treatment is allowed (2%)

Outcomes: subjective outcome measures are used and accurately described (2%); semi-objectives measures are used (2%); objective outcome measures are used (2%)

Sample size: how the sample size was determined is reported (3%)

Randomisation: allocation is randomized (2%), method used to generate the random allocation sequence is described (4%); details of restriction are reported (1%)

Allocation concealment: mechanism used to implement the random allocation sequence and to conceal the sequence until intervention is described (2%)

Implementation: it is reported who generated the random allocation sequence, who enrolled participants, and who assigned participants to the interventions (1%)

Blinding: blinding is present (2%) with description of who was blinded after assignment to interventions and how blinding was performed (2%)

Placebo: a placebo was used (2%)

Statistical methods: statistical methods are accurately described (5%)

Results (30/100)

Flux of participants: the numbers of participants who were eligible, included or excluded, randomly assigned, received intended treatment, lost to follow up and analyzed for the primary outcome are described (2%) in a flow chart or table (2%), reasons are explained (2%) and less than 20 % of patients are lost to follow up (2%)

Recruitment: dates defining the periods of recruitment and follow-up are reported (3%)

Baseline data: a table showing baseline demographic characteristics for each group is presented with treated and control groups similar at the start of the trial (8%)

Subjects analyzed: it is reported whether the results were analyzed by Intention to Treat or Per Protocol (3%)

Results: results for each group were accurately described (3%)

Analyses: results of any analyses are explained (2%); the effect size and clinical significance are reported (1%)

Risks: all important harms or unintended effects in each group are adequately explained (2%)

Discussion (15/100)

Limitations: trial limitations, sources of potential bias, imprecision, and, if relevant, multiplicity of analyses, are addressed (5%)

Generalizability: generalizability (external validity, applicability) of the trial findings is discussed (5%)

Interpretation: interpretation consistent with results, balancing benefits and harms, and considering other relevant evidence, are provided (5%)

Additional information (3/100)

Funding: funding sources and other supports (for example pharmaceutical firms) (1%) are mentioned, and absence or presence of conflicts of interest is declared (2%)

Adapted from Vandeweerd JM, Coisnon C, Clegg P, et al. Efficacy of nutraceuticals for the treatment of osteoarthritis: what can we learn from a systematic review? J Vet Intern Med 2012, in press.

when the number of studies and the number of tested animals are adequate. All other situations are considered inadequate.

In step 3, the consistency of results is assessed—that is, whether conclusions of different studies about one substance highlight a similar effect, through either an improvement or an absence of effect. Consistency is adequate when all studies indicate a similar effect of treatment. When the effects of one intervention are studied in only one trial, the consistency cannot be evaluated.

In step 4, it is considered whether the studies demonstrate a statistically significant effect or not (change in measured outcome).

Step 5 aims to obtain a global strength of evidence provided by the studies on a given intervention (ie, whether there are low or strong indications for its clinical use). Evidence is strong when there is adequate quantity and consistency of high- or intermediate-quality studies demonstrating a significant effect. They are low in all other situations.

Reporting the results clearly is also important to ensure transparency. Usually tabular summaries are used to describe groups, interventions, and outcomes of the different studies. Quality assessment can be reported in tables or graphs.

STATISTICAL ANALYSIS OF DATA

When it is possible, a graphical presentation of the outcomes of individual studies is provided under the form of a point estimate plot with a 95% confidence interval (CI) for each study (known as a "forest plot").[3,12] Statistical tools can also be used to describe and analyze the heterogeneity between studies.

These graphic representations are possible only if comparable data are available in all studies, which is not the most common situation in veterinary medicine. It is therefore important to try to obtain a consensus on the variables of interest in every area of research. For example, in studies focusing on mastitis therapy, it could be difficult to compare directly the rate of clinical cure versus the cows' bacteriological cure versus the udder quarters' bacteriological cure.

In the left side of a forest plot (**Fig. 2**), we usually find the list of the publications sorted by date of publication. In the right side, a square indicates the value of the effect measure that was investigated in the study. The horizontal line crossing the square indicates the 95% confidence interval around the measure of the effect. The vertical line corresponds to the absence of effect. If the effect measure is an odd ratio or a relative risk, the absence of effect due to the factor under study corresponds to the value of 1. For example, if a relative risk equals 1, it means that the risk that an event takes place (to die, for example) in case of exposition to the factor under study

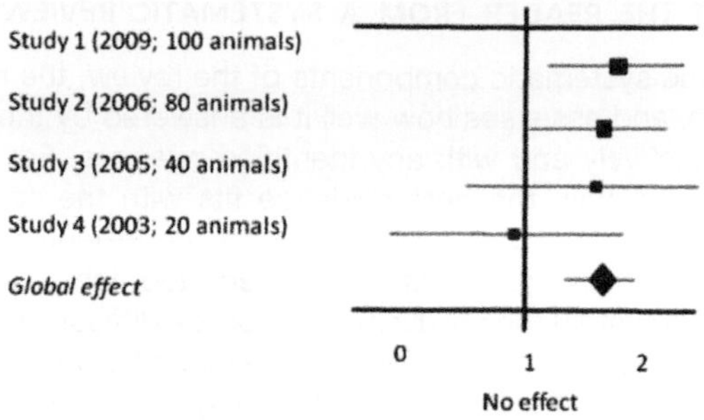

Fig. 2. Forest plot.

equals the risk that it does take place in absence of exposition to that factor. It is therefore possible to evaluate the significance of the effect for every study by looking at the extent of the confidence interval relatively to that vertical line. A confidence interval of 95% around the effect measure between A and B indicates that there is 95% of chance that the true value of the effect measure is situated between A and B. If the confidence interval includes the value of 1, the effect is statistically nonsignificant, as there is a chance that the true value of the effect is equal to 1, which corresponds to the absence of effect. In **Fig. 2**, the results of study 1 and 2 are statistically significant, but they are not for studies 3 and 4.

It is also sometimes possible to obtain a global effect (summary estimator) which is usually indicated by a lozenge at the bottom of the forest plot. In **Fig. 2**, we can see that the global effect is significant, as the value 1 is not included in its confidence interval. For calculating the global effect, every study has a weight that is proportional to the number of cases enrolled in the study. It is also of interest to note that adding multiple studies for meta-analysis decrease the 95% confidence interval of the effect showing a more precise estimate of the true effect. **Fig. 3** shows that the heterogeneity of studies can also be easily assessed using a forest plot. Heterogeneity is present when we find some studies on both sides of the vertical line showing that the nature of the effect was different in these studies.

However, it remains important to understand that meta-analysis, despite its visual interest using Forest plot, could only be soundly interpreted if the quality and risk of bias of the included studies have been previously thoroughly appraised.

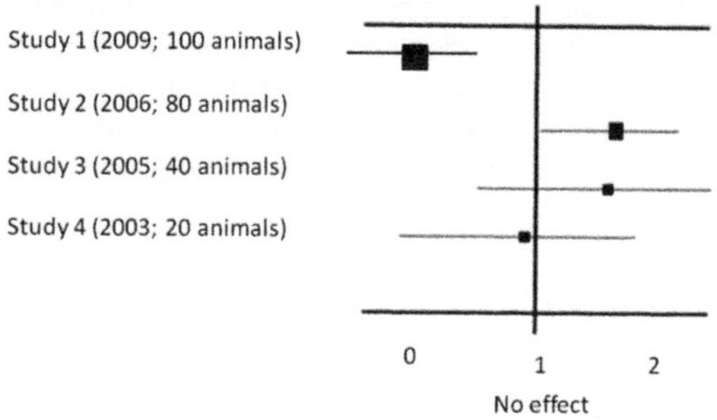

Fig. 3. Forest plot and heterogeneity of studies.

WHAT CAN EXPECT THE READER FROM A SYSTEMATIC REVIEW?

Having completed the systematic components of the review, the reviewer returns to the original question, and assesses how well it is answered by the current evidence, discussing data objectively and with any identified nuances. For the reader, it is a question of considering how the best evidence fits with the case in the clinically answerable question. For the reader, several points are essential.

First, due to the exhaustive data that may be reported, tables are not always user friendly, and reading a systematic review may become a difficult and tedious task. The results should be clearly reported so that the reader can quickly identify the best studies, rapidly confirm that adequate methodology has been applied to assess quality, and identify possible bias that would weaken the conclusion of some studies. **Box 1** can be useful to indicate these strengths and weaknesses of every article that is included in the final systematic review.[10] The way results are reported may provide transparency by providing the raw data (the references of the publications included in the review), the outcome measures (the question items), and the scores for every question item, thus allowing readers to repeat the review and compare their personal rating to those reported by the reviewers. **Box 1** also draws attention to important methodologic issues such as randomization, allocation concealment, sequence allocation, blinding, flux of participants, periods of recruitment and follow-up, baseline data, concept of "effect size," power of studies, sample size, and the use of objective outcome measures. As such, it is an interesting training tool to critical appraisal of literature.

Second, besides such methodologic aspects, there are other elements that may influence the evaluation of interventions. Varying and uncontrolled composition of the marketed product, combination of drugs, and wide range of dosages and durations of treatment are possible confounders. A clear description of interventions should therefore appear in an additional box or table.

Third, as veterinary practitioners have limited time to consult the literature, it is certain that they will be able to read the full paper of a systematic review. Therefore, abstracts should be accurately written so that they include useful and relevant information that could be quickly consulted in the summaries provided by free web database like PubMed.

SUMMARY

Bovine veterinarians need to base their clinical decisions on the best scientific evidence. Due to lack of time, the relevant information should be available in a structured and summarized publication, such as systematic reviews. These evaluate exhaustively the available literature regarding a specific clinical question and assess the quality of the studies, before choosing and discussing those that provide the best evidence to answer that question. Ideally, the results and the discussion should be reported in a practical and useful way for the practitioner. It is vital that every effort is made to design user friendly forms of systematic reviews. A structured abstract indicating briefly the material and methods, the results, and authors' conclusion is warranted to help the busy practitioner to have a quick look on the evidence gained by this approach. From a practical perspective, reviewing topics using the systematic review approach is a good way to assess the level of evidence supporting a treatment or vaccine efficacy, a feed additive, a diagnostic test, or a hormonal protocol. One issue for authors who want to do this exercise is that there is a lack of studies in many area of ruminant health compared with human health. Although this can be perceived as a limitation, veterinarians and scientists should design strategies to develop more systematic reviews. Besides the immediate scientific information that these provide, they may also help to assess future needs for clinical research in accurately identifying the gap of knowledge and to point future needs of veterinary research.

REFERENCES

1. Marr CM, Newton JR. Clinical evidence articles in Equine Veterinary Journal: progress since inception. Equine Vet J 2006;38:110–2.
2. Holmes MA. Philosophical foundations of evidence-based medicine for veterinary clinicians. J Am Vet Med Assoc 2009;235:1035–9.
3. Glasziou P, Irwig L, Bain C, et al. Systematic reviews in health care. Cambridge (UK): Cambridge University Press; 2001.
4. Lean IJ, Rabiee AR, Duffield TF, et al. Invited review: Use of meta-analysis in animal health and reproduction: methods and applications. J Dairy Sci 2009;92:3545–65.
5. Schulz KF, Altman DG, Moher D. CONSORT 2010 statement: Updated guidelines for reporting parallel group randomised trials. J Pharmacol Pharmacother 2010;1:100–7.
6. von Elm E, Altman DG, Egger M, et al. The Strengthening the Reporting of Observational Studies in Epidemiology (STROBE) statement: guidelines for reporting observational studies. Epidemiology 2007;18:800–4.
7. Fung AE, Palanki R, Bakri SJ, et al. Applying the CONSORT and STROBE statements to evaluate the reporting quality of neovascular age-related macular degeneration studies. Ophthalmology 2009;116:286–96.
8. Sargeant JM, O'Connor AM, Gardner IA, et al. The REFLECT statement: reporting guidelines for randomized controlled trials in livestock and food safety: explanation and elaboration. Food Prot 2010;73:579–603.
9. O'Connor A. Reporting guidelines for primary research: Saying what you did. Prev Vet Med 2010;97:144–9.
10. Vandeweerd JM, Coisnon C, Clegg P, et al. Efficacy of nutraceuticals for the treatment of osteoarthritis: what can we learn from a systematic review? J Vet Intern Med 2012, in press.
11. FDA/CFSAN. 2003. Guidance for industry and FDA: Interim evidence-based ranking for scientific data. Available at: http://www.fda.gov/ohrms/dockets/dockets/04q0072/04q-0072-pdn0001-05-FDA-vol5.pdf. Accessed January 10, 2010.
12. Fletcher RH, Fletcher SW. Clinical epidemiology: The essentials. 4th edition. Philadelphia: Lippincott Williams and Wilkins; 2005.

Evidence Related to the Use of Ancillary Drugs in Bovine Respiratory Disease (Anti-Inflammatory and Others): Are They Justified or Not?

David Francoz, DMV, DÉS, MSc[a,*], Sébastien Buczinski, Dr Vét, DÉS, MSc[a], Mike Apley, DVM, PhD[b]

KEYWORDS

- Ancillary drugs • Bovine respiratory disease
- Anti-inflammatory drugs • Immunomodulators • NSAIDs

Bovine respiratory disease (BRD) remains a major problem in dairy cattle,[1] cow-calf operations,[2] and the feedlot industry.[3] The major costs of this complex are due to mortality, treatment costs, and an adverse impact on growth, milk production, or average daily gain (ADG) of the affected animals.[4–6] Nonresponders or chronic animals can also maintain respiratory pathogens within the herd or the pen, thus potentially acting as a source of future BRD outbreaks.[7]

Since the etiology of BRD is complex and primarily associated with mixed infections of both viral and bacterial agents, classic recommendations concerning naturally occurring BRD treatment are based on systemic antimicrobial treatment.[8,9] Antimicrobial treatment can be used in cattle acutely affected by BRD but can also be used for control of BRD in cattle with a high risk of developing the disease.[9]

One of the major pathophysiologic consequences of BRD is lung damage caused by inflammatory cells, endotoxin release due to gram-negative bacteria, and cytokines that may lead to the classic signs of BRD: fever, depression, anorexia, and abnormal respiratory function.[10] Even if therapy is a success, chronic lung lesions are a common sequelae of BRD. Chronic lung lesions found at slaughter are associated with

The authors have nothing to disclose.

[a] Département des Sciences Cliniques, Faculté de Médecine Vétérinaire, St-Hyacinthe, Université de Montréal, CP 5000, J2S 7C6 Québec, Canada

[b] Department of Clinical Sciences, College of Veterinary Medicine, Kansas State University 111B Mosier Hall, Manhattan, KS 66506, USA

* Corresponding author.

E-mail address: david.francoz@umontreal.ca

Vet Clin Food Anim 28 (2012) 23–38
doi:10.1016/j.cvfa.2011.12.003
vetfood.theclinics.com
0749-0720/12/$ – see front matter

decreased performance of affected animals.[4,5] For these reasons the concomitant use of an anti-inflammatory drug (AID) has been recommended by some authors to decrease the severity of clinical symptoms,[11,12] increase appetite,[13] and decrease inflammation-induced lung damage,[14] thereby limiting the impact of BRD on weight gain or milk production. Decreasing clinical sign severity or their duration may also be viewed as a way to improve cattle welfare and therefore can be of interest from this perspective.

Transient or permanent depression of the immune system has also been documented as a predisposing factor for developing BRD. Immunosuppressed cattle are more susceptible to viral infection.[15,16] Virus-induced immunosuppression is also a predisposing factor for secondary bacterial infection.[17] For these reasons, several compounds have been used to improve immune function and recovery of cattle afflicted with BRD.[8]

Despite the theoretical potential of these different ancillary drugs to improve recovery of cattle affected by BRD, a summary of the scientific evidence concerning the efficacy of ancillary therapy is not available for naturally occurring BRD.

The objective of this article was therefore to conduct a systematic review concerning the efficacy of ancillary drugs for treating naturally occurring BRD concurrently with an antimicrobial.

MATERIAL AND METHODS

After consultation among the current authors, the Patient/Population, Intervention, Comparison, and Outcome of clinical importance (PICO) strategy was used. The clinical question we tried to answer was, In cattle with naturally occurring BRD, are there any beneficial effects of adding an ancillary drug to antimicrobial treatment? Parameters to be evaluated for a beneficial effect were rectal temperature, the relapse rate, failure of treatment, the short- to long-term ADG or feed efficiency, the lung lesions, and production data, all of which were considered between treated and untreated groups.

Search Strategy

In reference to the question, these keywords were selected by the authors: bovine respiratory disease; pneumonia; lung disease; steroids; dexamethasone; isoflupredone; NSAIDs; flunixin; meloxicam; acetylsalicylic acid; ketoprofen; antihistamines; tripelennamine; immunostimulants; interferon; levamisole; vitamin C; concurrent vaccination; cattle; calf; bovine; veterinary.

The initial web search was conducted independently by 2 of the authors using the database MEDLINE (1966–2010) and CAB abstract (1984–2010). The search did not include regulatory document databases, which may have included reports of trials conducted during the approval process and which were not subsequently published. No restrictions were applied. For the web search in PubMed, the equation used was: bovine respiratory disease or pneumonia or lung disease and (steroids or dexamethasone or isoflupredone or NSAIDs or flunixin or meloxicam or acetylsalicylic acid or ketoprofen or antihistamines or tripelennamine or immunostimulants or interferon or levamisole or vitamin C or concurrent vaccination) and (cattle or calf or bovine) and veterinary. A similar equation was used in the CAB abstract database: ("bovine respiratory disease" or "pneumonia" or "lung disease").mp. and ("steroids" or "dexamethasone" or "isoflupredone" or "NSAIDs" or "flunixin" or "meloxicam" or "acetylsalicylic acid" or "ketoprofen" or "antihistamines" or "tripelennamine" or "immunostimulants" or "interferon" or "levamisole" or "vitamin C" or "concurrent vaccination").mp and ("cattle" or "calf" or "bovine").mp.

Identification of Relevant Studies

Identification of relevant studies was performed independently by 2 of the authors. After the 2 datasets were obtained, the titles were checked for their pertinence in regard to objectives of the study. The abstract of the articles obtained were then assessed. If no abstract was available, the manuscripts were obtained and read. To be included in the review, studies must have involved the treatment of naturally occurring BRD with antibiotics with and without an ancillary drug. As a consequence, articles dealing with induced experimental models, the use of ancillary drugs for BRD prevention, studies assessing ancillary treatment without a control group (eg, 2 groups with different nonsteroidal anti-inflammatory drugs [NSAIDs] but no group without an NSAID), or studies dealing with different antimicrobial treatments in the treatment groups were rejected from further reviewing. The articles that were not published in English (read by all authors) or in French (read by SB and DF) were not kept for further analysis. All other references were extracted and fully screened by the authors. The lists of manuscripts obtained independently were then compared and a definitive list of manuscripts for critical appraisal was made.

Critical Appraisal of Selected Studies

The articles were assessed using a 100-point scoring version of the CONSORT 2010 checklist for information to include when reporting a randomized clinical trial (RCT)[18] (see article by Vandeweerd and colleagues elsewhere in this issue for further exploration of this topic). The score attributed to each study increased as the quality of the methodology increased and the risk of bias decreased. The 3 authors independently reviewed the articles, except for French published articles, which were reviewed by 2 of the authors (SB and DF), and then compared their score leading to a mean score of each article. The articles were then ranked based on their score. As previously described, article quality can be classified as high (score of more than 60%), moderate (score between 45% and 60%), and low (<45%) (see article by Vandeweerd and colleagues elsewhere in this issue for further exploration of this topic). For complete extraction and evaluation of studies' results, the articles must have been randomized, masked (blinded), and prospective (ie, RCT) and have appropriate statistics. Due to the difference of methodology and the outcomes used in the articles, it was not possible to assess the scientific evidence using meta-analysis and forest plots quantifying the extent of the effect on the outcome studied.

Data Extraction

The following general information on the manuscript was recorded: authors, journal, year of publication, potential conflict of interest (which generally means that the data were presented by researchers from the pharmaceutical company distributing the drug and/or the study was funded by the company producing the product), and country where the trial was performed. Data extracted on the methodology included randomization, masking, treatment regimen, population studied and group size, outcome parameters, as well as frequency of evaluation and duration of the study. Significant results involving rectal temperature, clinical signs, relapse or failure after treatment, mortality, production data (eg, ADG), and other potential effects of ancillary treatment were recorded.

RESULTS

Search Process and Identification of Relevant Studies

Only 15 articles met the initial criteria, 14 dealt with AIDs (12 NSAIDs, 1 steroidal anti-inflammatory drug [SAID], and 1 both SAID and NSAID) and 1 with immunomodulators.

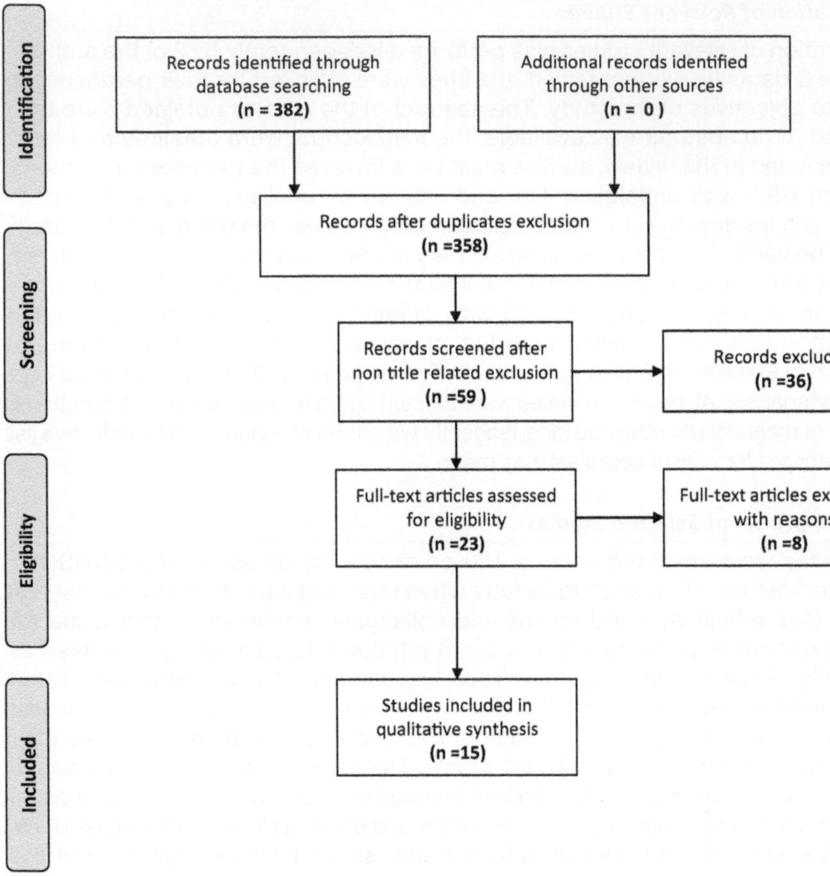

Fig. 1. Flow diagram indicating the data recording in systematic review on ancillary drugs treatment in naturally occurring BRD. (*From* Moher D, Liberati A, Tetzlaff J, et al. Preferred reporting items for systematic reviews and meta-analyses: the PRISMA statement. BMJ 2009;339:b2535; with permission.)[27]

The reviewing process and extraction of the data are described in **Fig. 1**. Briefly, 358 different articles were found using the search strategy previously mentioned. Among the 59 articles remaining after title exclusion, 36 were excluded for the following reasons: 2 were studies utilizing an experimental model, 3 were the same study presented 2 times in different journals or proceedings, 5 were reviews of literature or non related to the specific objectives of the present study, 7 were studies on prevention rather than treatment of BRD, and 19 were not in English or French. Following complete review of the manuscripts, 4 additional articles were excluded because there was no control group, 3 because different antibiotics were used, and finally 1 article was excluded because it could not be considered as an evaluation of an ancillary treatment.

Study Information and Evaluation

General information on the 15 included studies, their score based on the CONSORT assessment of the articles, as well as treatment regimens are presented in **Tables 1** and **2**.

Table 1
General information on the articles and CONSORT evaluation results

Ref.	Year of Publication	Country	Author(s) Affiliated With a Pharmaceutical Lab	Randomized	Blinded	*n*	Duration of the Study (d)	CONSORT Evaluation SB	DF	MA	Mean
Anti-inflammatory studies											
12	2003	USA	Yes	Yes	Yes	66	4–5	48	57	49	51
11	1994	France/Belgium	Yes	Yes[a]	Yes[a]	199	22	52	50	37	46
21	2005	Mexico	Yes	Yes	Yes	200	172	34	51	44	43
23	1986	Netherlands	No	Yes[a]	Yes[a]	23	7	51	39	30	40
20	2010	Turkey	No	Yes[a]	Yes[a]	80	15	27	43	37	36
13	2004	Turkey	No	NM	NM	40	3	31	36	29	32
28	2003	Poland	No	Yes[a]	NM	30	5	31	37	28	32
29	1994	UK	No	No[b]	No	119	46	34	25	25	28
22	2000	USA	Yes	Yes[a]	Yes[a]	52	35	27	27	25	26
30	1982	Romania	No	NM	NM	20/20	14/21	15	34	ND	24.5
31	1986	France	Yes	NM	Yes[a]	48	15	22	21	ND	21.5
32	2003	Poland	No	Yes[a]	NM	18	3	20	20	23	21
33	1988	UK	Yes	Yes[a]	No	97	151	23	18	ND	20.5
34	1986	France	Yes	Yes[a]	No	60	3	26	8	13	16
Immunomodulator studies											
19	1996	Poland	No	NM	NM	30	About 96	16	22	11	16

NM, not mentioned.
[a] No indication on how the randomization or the blinding was performed.
[b] NSAIDs were administered to every other head.

Table 2
Population studied and treatment regimen of the 15 included studies

Ref[a]	Population Studied	Antimicrobial (*n* Control Group)	AIDs (*n*)
51[12]	Mixed beef breed cattle (calves, 197 kg)	Ceftiofur (1.1 mg/kg, 3 doses, D0, 1, 2) (*n* = 17)	Flunixin meglumine (2.2 mg/kg, once D0) (*n* = 17) Ketoprofen (3 mg/kg, once D0) (*n* = 16) Carprofen (1.4 mg/kg, once D0) (*n* = 16)
46[11]	Mixed breed beef and dairy cattle (calves 209 ± 90 kg)	Oxytetracycline (20 mg/kg, once, D0) (*n* = 70)	Tolfenamic acid (2 mg/kg, once, D0) (*n* = 65) Tolfenamic acid (2 mg/kg, twice, D0, 2) (*n* = 64)
43[21]	Brahman and crossed-Brahman (calves, 230 kg)	Oxytetracycline (20 mg/kg, once D0) (*n* = 100)	Meloxicam (0.5 mg/kg, once, D0) (*n* = 100)
40[23]	Dairy cattle (calves, 3–8 mo)	Oxytetracycline (10 mg/kg, 3 doses, D0, 1, 2) (*n* = 10)	Flunixin meglumine (2 mg/kg, twice, D0, 1) (*n* = 13)
36[20]	Holstein (calves, 3–5 mo; 60–155 kg)	Tulathromycin (2.5 mg/kg, once D0) (*n* = 20)	Diclofenac (2.5 mg/kg, once D0) (*n* = 30) Flunixin meglumine (2.2 mg/kg, 3 doses D0, 1, 2) (*n* = 30)
32[13]	Cattle (6 mo–3 y; 250–630 kg)	Tilmicosin (10 mg/kg, once, D0) (*n* = 20)	Carprofen (1.4 mg/kg, once, D0) (*n* = 20)
32[28]	Black and White Lowland breed (calves, 1–2 mo; 76 kg)	Oxytetracycline (20 mg/kg, once, D0) (*n* = 10)	Meloxicam (0.5 mg/kg, twice D0, 2) (*n* = 10) Flumethasone (0.03 mg/kg, twice, D0, 2) (*n* = 10)
28[29]	Mixed Breed Beef cattle (calves)	Tilmicosin (10 mg/kg, once D0) (*n* = 61)	Flunixin meglumine (2.2 mg/kg, once, D0) (*n* = 58)
26[22]	Stockers calves (180–240 kg)	Tilmicosin (10 mg/kg, once, D0) (*n* = 26)	Flunixin meglumine (2.2 mg/kg, once, D0) (*n* = 26)
24.5[30]	Simmental (calves, 1 mo)	Chloramphenicol (NA) + ascorbic acid (500 mg/calf/day, NA) (*n* = 10)	Aspirin (100 mg/kg, BID, 14 days D0–13) (*n* = 10)
	Simmental (calves, 2 mo)	Chloramphenicol (NA) + sulfamides (NA) (*n* = 5)	Aspirin (135 mg/kg, BID, 21 days) + bromhexin (1 g/calf, BID, 21 days) (*n* = 9) Aspirin (135 mg/kg, BID, 5 days then 200 mg/kg, BID, 16 days) + bromhexin (1 g/calf, BID, 5 days then 1.5 g/calf, BID, 16 days) (*n* = 6)

(*continued on next page*)

Table 2
(*continued*)

Ref[a]	Population Studied	Antimicrobial (*n* Control Group)	AIDs (*n*)
21.5[31]	Salers (calves, 280 kg)	Oxytetracycline (5 mg/kg, 5 doses, D0, 1, 2, 3, 4) + chloramphenicol (10 mg/kg, 5 doses, D0, 1, 2, 3, 4) + DMSO (5 days) (*n* = 6)	Prednisolone acetate (0.5 mg/kg, 5 doses D0, 1, 2, 3, 4) (*n* = 28) Prednisolone acetate (0.5 mg/kg, 2 doses, D0, 1) (*n* = 6) Methylprednisolone (0.4 mg/kg, 2 doses, D0, 1) (*n* = 8)
21[32]	Black and White Lowland breed (calves, 2–2.5 mo, 87 kg)	Oxytetracycline (20 mg/kg, once, D0) (*n* = 6)	Meloxicam (0.5 mg/kg, once, D0) (*n* = 9) Flunixin meglumine (2.2 mg/kg, once D0) (*n* = 3)
20.5[33]	Mixed Crossed Breed cattle (4–7 mo)	Oxytetracycline (10 mg/kg, 3 doses, D0, 1, 2) (*n* = 48)	Flunixin meglumine (2 mg/kg, 3 doses, D0, 1, 2) (*n* = 49)
16[34]	Mixed Crossed Beef Breed cattle (214–345 kg)	Spiramycin (100 000 UI/kg, twice, D0 and 2) (*n* = 30)	Ketoprofen (3 mg/kg, 3 doses, D0, 1, 2) (*n* = 30)
16[19]	Lowland Black-white breed (calves, 80 kg)	Ampicillin (about 37.5–50 mg/kg, once, D0) (*n* = 10)	Vetokhel (1 mL, twice, D0 and 5) (*n* = 10)

[a] Mean CONSORT evaluation score and reference number.

The different AIDs evaluated included flunixin meglumine (7 studies), meloxicam (3 studies), carprofen, tolfenamic acid, and ketoprofen (2 studies each), diclofenac (1 study), and the corticosteroids flumethasone, prednisolone acetate, and methylprednisolone. The only immunomodulator evaluated was Vetokelh sub D4 (*Bacillus subtilis* D4; Sanum Kehlbeck).[19]

For the same molecule, the dosage and number of administrations may differ between the different studies. Additionally, the population studied and the number of animals included differed greatly between studies (**Table 2**). Five studies were considered to be of short or very short duration (<7 days), 6 of middle duration (<45 days), and 2 of long duration (151 and 172 days). All these points make comparison between studies difficult.

Only 2 studies (mean score of 51[12] and 46[11]) had a consort evaluation above 45, indicating an overall low level of validity and reliability of the manuscripts. Only 6 studies were randomized and masked,[11,12,20–23] but the process for randomization or blinding was explained in only 2 studies.[12,21] Interestingly, 7 of the 15 studies had at least one author affiliated with a company that distributed the ancillary drug tested and none had declared potential conflict of interests. It should also be noted that in all of these studies, the authors concluded there was a significant effect of the ancillary treatment for at least one outcome parameter compared with the control group or with other ancillary drugs.

Study Results

Outcomes of interest that were evaluated and significant results of the 6 studies that were randomized and blinded are summarized in **Tables 3** and **4**. Four of these

Table 3
Outcome of interest evaluated and the frequency of the evaluations of the 6 randomized controlled trials concerning the use of NSAIDs as ancillary treatment for BRD

Ref[a]	Outcome of Interest Evaluated	Frequency
51[12]	Rectal temperature	H0, 2, 4, 6, 12, 24, 48, and 72
	Clinical score	D0, 1, 2, and 3
	Clinical success (failure)	D3
	Lung lesions score	D4 or 5
46[11]	Rectal temperature	D0, 1, 2, 3, and 4
	Clinical index score	D0, 1, 2, 3, and 4
	Weight gain	D0 and D21
	Relapses	D5 to 21
43[21]	Rectal temperature	D0, D1, 2, 3, and 7
	Clinical index score	D0, D1, 2, 3, and 7
	Relapse	D3, 7, and until slaughter
	Lung lesions score	Slaughter
	Weight	D0, 7, 35, 70, 105, and 1 D before slaughter (D170)
40[23]	Rectal temperature	D0/H0 and H4, 1 (and 4 hours after treatment), 2, 4, and 6
	Respiratory rate	D0/H0 and H4, 1 (and 4 hours after treatment), 2, 4, and 6
	PaO_2	D0/H0 and H4, 1 (and 4 hours after treatment), 2, 4, and 6
36[20]	Rectal temperature	D0, 1, 2, 3, 7, and 14
	Clinical index score	D0, 1, 2, 3, 7, and 14
	Improvement (failure)	D7 and 14
26[22]	Treatment failure	D2
	Treatment success	D2
	Relapse	D2 to D35
	Weight	Throughout the study (35 days)
	Cost of treatment	Throughout the study (35 days)

Frequency is reported as either study hour (H) or day (D).
[a] Mean CONSORT evaluation score and reference number.

studies used clinical index scoring systems for assessment of clinical improvement, all of which were different.

Effect on fever and clinical signs
The only consistent positive effect of NSAID treatment was a more rapid decrease in rectal temperature in the early follow-up period (**Table 4**). On the other hand, no beneficial effects of NSAID treatment were observed related to clinical signs at the end of any of the studies.

Effect on relapse rate, treatment failures, and mortality
Despite the fact that 5 of 6 RCTs measured relapse rate and treatment failure, NSAID treatment significantly decreased the proportion of treatment failures or relapses in

Table 4
Main significant results of the 6 RCTs concerning the use of NSAIDs as ancillary treatment for BRD

		Clinical Signs		Relapse/Failure		Mortality Reported in the Study		
Ref[a]	Faster Temperature Drop	Initial Benefits	Benefit at the End of the Study	Yes/No	Any Difference in Treatment Groups	Yes/No	Any Difference in Treatment Groups	Other NSAID Benefits
51[12]	Yes	No	No	Yes all groups	No	Yes in carprofen group on D1	No	Decrease lung consolidation for flunixin group
46[11]	NM	Yes for tolfenamic acid twice	No	Yes all groups	No	No	NA	No (no difference in weight gain)
43[21]	Yes	No	No	Yes all groups	No	No	NA	Increased weight gain Decrease lung consolidation
40[23]	Yes[b]	NM	No	NM	NM	Yes in flunixin group	No	No
36[20]	Yes	Yes	No	Yes all groups	No	No	NA	Decrease respiratory rate
26[22]	NM	NM	NM	Yes	Yes[c]	No	NA	(no difference in weight gain or treatment cost)

NM, not mentioned; NA, not available.
[a] Mean CONSORT evaluation score and reference number.
[b] Significant decrease at 4 hours post-treatment only compared to pre-treatment temperatures; the control group decrease was not significant at 4 hours.
[c] The success of treatment was based on decreased temperature under 39.4°C at 48 hours; no relapses were observed.

only 1 of the 5 studies.[22] However, the definitions of *success* and *failure* may be questionable in this particular study since the success was defined 48 hours after initial treatment with tilmicosin phosphate and flunixin meglumin, rather than 72 hours, and since any animal with a rectal temperature of 103°F (39.4°C) or higher was classified as a failure based on temperature alone.

The NSAID treatment did not have any impact on mortality in the 2 studies that reported these data.[12,22] However, these 2 studies had low numbers of animals per group and no power analysis calculation for the magnitude of difference that the study could detect was provided.

Effects on average daily gain or body weight and lung lesions

The NSAID effect on weight gain was only assessed in 3 RCTs,[11,21,22] No difference was found for ADG over a 35-day period in a study comparing tilmicosin phosphate to tilmicosin phosphate and flunixin meglumine.[22] By contrast, a study in Mexico showed that ADG was higher when assessed at 70, 105, and 172 days after BRD treatment using oxytetracycline and meloxicam versus oxytetracycline and a saline placebo.[21] In this study, the carcass weight and ADG after slaughter were increased compared with the control group.

Different NSAIDs were compared in 2 studies. A significantly faster decrease in rectal temperature was observed with diclofenac in comparison with flunixin meglumin (on study days 0 and 2),[20] and with ketoprofen and flunixin meglumin in comparison with carprofen (at post treatment hours 2 and 4).[12] Decreased lung consolidation was observed with flunixin meglumin but not with ketoprofen and carpofen.[12]

Decreased lung consolidation was attributed to meloxicam when used with oxytetracycline in the only other study to evaluate consolidation.[21]

Cost and cost-benefit of treatment were evaluated in only one study[22] and no difference between groups was observed; however, the complete data were not available.

Outcomes of interest, significant results, and the limitations of the 8 non–RCTs concerning the use of AIDs in BRD are summarized in **Tables 5** and **6**. A beneficial effect on weight was reported in the unique study dealing with the use of an immunomodulator in BRD.[19] However, the reliability and validity of the study are questionable as indicated by the lowest consort evaluation score.

DISCUSSION

The main objective of this systematic review was to evaluate ancillary treatments that may be beneficial in the treatment of BRD. Since the etiology of BRD is complex and multifactorial, it is necessary to have well-organized, published RCTs for clinicians to make decisions related to including or excluding ancillary therapies for BRD. The results reported here demonstrate that only 6 RCTs are available in the published literature for the evaluation of ancillary BRD treatment regimens in relation to negative controls. Among them, only NSAID administration as an adjunct to antimicrobial treatment had been studied. However, the systemic evaluation of these 6 studies using a scored version of the CONSORT table was under 60% for all studies and under 45% for 4, raising the issue of the validity and reliability of these studies. In this context, it is difficult to conclude with a high degree of conviction on the potential beneficial effects of these NSAID treatments. On the other hand, the CONSORT table used was developed for human clinical trials and not for veterinary medicine, which could have lowered the score of the included studies.

Indications concerning the inclusion criteria, the number of animals that could be included, the number finally included, and the reason of exclusion of other animals

Table 5
Outcome of interest evaluated and the frequency of the evaluations of the 8 non-RCTs concerning the use of NSAIDs as ancillary treatment for BRD

Ref[a]	Outcome of Interest Evaluated	Frequency
32[13]	Clinical score	H0, 6, 12, 24, 48, and 72
	Rectal temperature	H0, 6, 12, 24, 48, and 72
32[28]	Rectal temperature	D0, 1, 2, 3, and 4
	Clinical index score	D0, 1, 2, 3, and 4
	Mortality	D0, 1, 2, 3, and 4
28[29]	Rectal temperature	NA
	Relapse	NA
24.5[30]	General condition	Daily, 14/21 days (?)
	Rectal temperature	Daily, 14/21 days (?)
	Weight gain	D0 and D13/D20
21[32]	Rectal temperature	D0 and 2
20.5[33]	Rectal temperature	D0, 1, 2, 10, and 20
	Weight	D0, 10, 20, 30, 40, 60, 90, and 150
	Relapse/failure	Throughout the study (?)
21.5[31]	Rectal temperature	D0 to 4
	General clinical score	D0 to 4
	Relapse	D4 to 9
16[34]	Rectal temperature	H0, 3, 8, 24, 27, 32, 48, 51, 56, and 72

[a] Mean CONSORT evaluation score and reference number.

were not commonly mentioned. Most of the studies reviewed in this study lack information as to the methods for performing randomization and blinding. Some authors presented their study as an RCT despite the lack of evidence in the article to this effect. For example, it is not clear how animals could be randomly allocated to 1 of 2 treatment groups and a control group when the final number of study animals were 30 in both treatment groups and 20 for control group.[20] An intentionally unbalanced design should be described in the methods. Also, it must be explained in the methods how a study can be double blind when clinicians assessing the animals are administering the drugs via different routes depending on the treatment group without any placebo injection.[20]

Data on specifics of parameters evaluated, as well as procedures for study animal follow-up, were frequently missing or incomplete. Finally, conflicts of interest, even if obviously present, were not mentioned. It can be noted that when comparing different NSAIDs, trials in which one of the authors was from a pharmaceutical company always pointed at a significant difference in favor of the NSAID distributed by the company. All these points together explain the weak score of the studies. The generally low number of animals per group, the absence of a clear null hypothesis and pre–study power-size calculation were also limiting factors contributing to the low scores from the reviewers. For these reasons, the authors propose that further research performed on that topic should be done according to the highest standards for reporting controlled trials (CONSORT statement).[18]

Table 6
Nonrandomized or blinding control trial studies on AID use in BRD: findings and concerns on internal validity of the studies that were assessed

		Clinical Signs		Relapse/Failure		Mortality Reported in the Study			
Ref[a]	Faster Temperature Drop	Initial Benefits	Benefit at the End of the Study	Yes/No	Any Difference in Treatment Groups	Yes/No	Any Difference in Treatment Groups	Other NSAI Benefits	Concerns (Other Than Blinding or Randomization)
32[13]	Yes	No	No	NM	NM	No	NA	Decrease respiratory rate	No explanation on clinical score
32[28]	Yes	Yes	No	NM	NM	No	NA	No	Inclusion criteria unclear, no definition of cure/failure
21[32]	Yes[b]	NM	NM	NM	NM	No	NA	No	Control group had a mean rectal temperature lower than other group on D0, no data other than temperature
28[29]	No	NM	NM	Yes all groups	No	No	NA	No	One farm outbreak (field study)
24.5[30]	No	Yes	NM	NM	NM	No	NA	Decrease respiratory rate and increase weight gain (only descriptive data)	Study design, no statistical analysis

16[34]	Yes	NM	NM	NM	NM	No	NA	No	No inclusion criteria, no data other than rectal temperature
20.5[33]	NM	NM	NM	Yes	Yes	No	No	Increased weight gain	No inclusion criteria, no definition of relapse or failure
21.5[31]	NM	Yes for prednisolone acetate groups	Yes for prednisolone acetate for 5 days	Yes all groups except prednisolone 5 days	No	No	No	No	No inclusion criteria

NM, not mentioned; NA, not available.
[a] Mean CONSORT evaluation score and reference number.
[b] Significant decrease from D0 on D2 but temperature was not different from the control group.

One additional difficulty when assessing the results obtained in the presented studies was that they cannot be easily compared. Most of these studies had a low external validity. Differences in the studied population, the treatment regimen and the outcome parameters evaluated, and their frequency may explain some of the differences observed between the studies. As an example, none of these studies used the same clinical index scoring system. Overweighting of the rectal temperature in a composite score may bias the overall score, and therefore the conclusions related to overall clinical response. This could explain why a better score was observed in a group where rectal temperature is decreased due to effect of NSAIDs rather than effect on the respiratory signs and appetite. For these reasons it is difficult to clearly assess the effect of NSAIDs on parameters other than fever.

The combination of an NSAID with an antimicrobial for treatment of BRD has become a common practice over the past decade, at least for individual cases.[14,24] Their use in the treatment of BRD is based on their analgesic, antipyretic, and anti-inflammatory properties. They are expected to reduce the rectal temperature and abnormal clinical signs, thereby returning the animal to a normal appetite more quickly. Additionally, their anti-inflammatory properties may decrease the lung lesions remaining after the acute phase of BRD, for which lesions remaining at slaughter have be associated with decreased productivity.[5,25] Based on these considerations, animals treated with antimicrobials and NSAIDs are expected to return to productivity more quickly and to have higher production performance (higher weight gain or milk production). The faster drop in rectal temperature was observed in the early phase of all the studies. However, the faster normalization of clinical signs expected was not consistent among the reviewed studies. Lung consolidation was evaluated in only 2 studies and both demonstrated a positive effect of NSAID administration. Unfortunately, higher production performance evaluated by increased weight gain was only evaluated in 3 studies[11,21,22] and results were inconsistent, with only 1[21] of these studies reporting increased long-term weight gain for BRD cases treated with NSAIDs.

With all of these points taken together, we can conclude that the administration of NSAIDs as an ancillary treatment to BRD causes a more rapid decrease in rectal temperature of the animals without beneficial effects at the end of the treatment on clinical signs. The data also suggest that NSAIDs may decrease lung lesions at the end of the feeding period, but data are either lacking or inconsistent to conclude a potential positive effect on the productivity of treated animals and, consequently, on the positive cost-benefits of such treatments. However, one could argue that the initial benefits of NSAIDs may be significant from an animal welfare perspective. The inconsistency of the results concerning the improvements in clinical signs for animals treated with NSAIDs for BRD may mitigate this argument.

SAIDs are other potential AIDs that can be used in the treatment of BRD. However, because of their immunosuppressive effects their use is controversial and has been contraindicated.[24,26] SAIDs were involved in only 2 reviewed studies; both had serious limitations making conclusion impossible. Consequently, to date it is impossible to know if the potential benefits of SAIDs overwhelmed their potential deleterious expected effects in the treatment of BRD.

SUMMARY

In conclusion, scarce relevant information is actually available on the use of ancillary treatment in BRD other than NSAIDs. However, even studies on NSAIDs lack consistent reliability and validity. Well-designed RCTs of long duration are necessary to support conclusions related to the actual consequences of NSAID treatment.

These studies should include short-term data (temperature, clinical improvement, relapse, or failure to treatment) as well as long-term data (productivity parameters, cost-benefit measurements). In addition, standardization and validation of clinical index scores are also necessary in order to make meta-analyses of the studies possible.

REFERENCES

1. Gorden PJ, Plummer P. Control, management, and prevention of bovine respiratory disease in dairy calves and cows. Vet Clin North Am Food Anim Pract 2010;26:243–59.
2. Stokka GL. Prevention of respiratory disease in cow/calf operations. Vet Clin North Am Food Anim Pract 2010;26:229–41.
3. Smith RA. North American cattle marketing and bovine respiratory disease (BRD). Anim Health Res Rev 2009;10:105–8.
4. Schneider MJ, Tait RG Jr, Busby WD, et al. An evaluation of bovine respiratory disease complex in feedlot cattle: impact on performance and carcass traits using treatment records and lung lesion scores. J Anim Sci 2009;87:1821–7.
5. Wittum TE, Woollen NE, Perino LJ, et al. Relationships among treatment for respiratory tract disease, pulmonary lesions evident at slaughter, and rate of weight gain in feedlot cattle. J Am Vet Med Assoc 1996;209:814–8.
6. van der Fels-Klerx HJ, Sorensen JT, Jalvingh AW, et al. An economic model to calculate farm-specific losses due to bovine respiratory disease in dairy heifers. Prev Vet Med 2001;51:75–94.
7. Maunsell FP, Donovan GA. Mycoplasma bovis infections in young calves. Vet Clin North Am Food Anim Pract 2009;25:139–77, vii.
8. Apley M. Antimicrobials and BRD. Anim Health Res Rev 2009;10:159–61.
9. Edwards TA. Control methods for bovine respiratory disease for feedlot cattle. Vet Clin North Am Food Anim Pract 2010;26:273–84.
10. Griffin D, Chengappa MM, Kuszak J, et al. Bacterial pathogens of the bovine respiratory disease complex. Vet Clin North Am Food Anim Pract 2010;26:381–94.
11. Deleforge J, Thomas E, Davot JL, et al. A field evaluation of the efficacy of tolfenamic acid and oxytetracycline in the treatment of bovine respiratory disease. J Vet Pharmacol Ther 1994;17:43–7.
12. Lockwood PW, Johnson JC, Katz TL. Clinical efficacy of flunixin, carprofen and ketoprofen as adjuncts to the antibacterial treatment of bovine respiratory disease. Vet Rec 2003;152:392–4.
13. Elitok B, Elitok OM. Clinical efficacy of carprofen as an adjunct to the antibacterial treatment of bovine respiratory disease. J Vet Pharmacol Ther 2004;27:317–20.
14. Van De Weerdt ML, Lekeux P. Modulation of lung inflammation in the control of bovine respiratory disease. Bovine Pract 1997;31:19–30.
15. Taylor JD, Fulton RW, Lehenbauer TW, et al. The epidemiology of bovine respiratory disease: what is the evidence for predisposing factors? Can Vet J;51:1095–102.
16. Taylor JD, Fulton RW, Lehenbauer TW, et al. The epidemiology of bovine respiratory disease: what is the evidence for preventive measures? Can Vet J 2010;51:1351–9.
17. Ridpath J. The contribution of infections with bovine viral diarrhea viruses to bovine respiratory disease. Vet Clin North Am Food Anim Pract 2010;26:335–48.
18. Moher D, Hopewell S, Schulz KF, et al. CONSORT 2010 explanation and elaboration: updated guidelines for reporting parallel group randomised trials. BMJ 2010;340:c869.

19. Czernomysy-Furowicz D, Furowicz AJ. Comparison of therpaeutic effectiveness of immunomodulator Vetokehl Sub D4 (Sanum-Kehlbeck) and ampicillin in treatment of bronchopneumonia enzootica catarrhalis vitulorum. Sci Agri Bohem 1996;27:29–37.
20. Guzel M, Karakurum MC, Durgut R, et al. Clinical efficacy of diclofenac sodium and flunixin meglumine as adjuncts to antibacterial treatment of respiratory disease of calves. Aust Vet J 2010;88:236–9.
21. Friton GM, Cajal C, Ramirez-Romero R. Long-term effects of meloxicam in the treatment of respiratory disease in fattening cattle. Vet Rec 2005;156:809–11.
22. Hellwig DH, Kegley EB, Johnson Z, et al. Flunixine meglumine as adjunct therapy for bovine respiratory disease in stocker cattle. AAES Res Ser 2000;478:10–2.
23. Verhoeff J, Wierda A, van Vulpen C, et al. Flunixin meglumine in calves with natural bovine respiratory syncytial virus infection. Vet Rec 1986;118:14–6.
24. Fajt V, Lechtenberg K. Using anti-inflammatory drugs in the treatment of bovine respiratory disease. Large Anim Pract 1998;19:34–9.
25. Gardner BA, Dolezal HG, Bryant LK, et al. Health of finishing steers: effects on performance, carcass traits, and meat tenderness. J Anim Sci 1999;77:3168–75.
26. Barragry T. Treatment of pneumonia in growing stock. Irish Vet J 1997;50:435–41.
27. Moher D, Liberati A, Tetzlaff J, et al. Preferred reporting items for systematic reviews and meta-analyses: the PRISMA statement. BMJ 2009;339:b2535.
28. Bednarek D, Zdzisinska B, Kondracki M, et al. Effect of steroidal and non-steroidal anti-inflammatory drugs in combination with long-acting oxytetracycline on non-specific immunity of calves suffering from enzootic bronchopneumonia. Vet Microbiol 2003;96:53–67.
29. Scott PR. Field study of undifferentiated respiratory disease in housed beef calves. Vet Rec 1994;134:325–7.
30. Ghergariu S, Danielescu N, Pop AI, et al. Essais thérapeutiques avec l'aspirine dans les maladies respiratoires du veau. Rec Méd Vét 1982;158:355–62.
31. Espinasse J, Allaire R, Raynaud JP, et al. Corticothérapie associée à l'antibiothérapie dans les bronchopneumonies infectieuses enzootiques des jeunes bovins—BPIE. Résultats cliniques. Bovine Pract 1986;21:59–61.
32. Bednarek D, Zdzisinska B, Kondracki M, et al. A comparative study of the effects of meloxicam and flunixin meglumine (NSAIDs) as adjunctive therapy on interferon and tumor necrosis factor production in calves suffering from enzootic bronchopneumonia. Pol J Vet Sci 2003;6:109–15.
33. Haas V, de Abric JL, Anderson DB, et al. Intérêt de l'association d'un anti-inflammatoire non stéroidien (AINS), la flunixine méglumine, a un antibiotique dans le traitement d'une pneumonie chez le veau. Mal Respir Jeunes Bovins 1988;219–21.
34. Longo F, Consalvi PJ, van Gool F. Antipyretic effect of ketoprofen in the treatment of respiratory diseases in cattle. In: Proceedings 18th World Buiatrics Congress: 26th Congress of the Italian Association of Buiatrics, Bologna, Italy, August 29–September 2, 1994. Volume 2. Bologna (Italy): Societa Italiana di Buiatria; 1994. p. 1343–6.

Systematic Review: What is the Best Antibiotic Treatment for *Staphylococcus aureus* Intramammary Infection of Lactating Cows in North America?

Jean-Philippe Roy, DVM, MSc[a,*], Greg Keefe, DVM, MSc, MBA[b]

KEYWORDS

- Systematic review • *Staphylococcus aureus* • Bovine
- Mastitis • Treatment • Antibiotic • Lactation

Staphylococcus aureus is still one of the most prevalent pathogens causing intramammary infections (IMI) in dairy cattle worldwide.[1–6] *S aureus* is typically recognized as a cause of chronic subclinical infections with elevation of somatic cell count (SCC) but may also cause clinical mastitis.[7] In fact, it is the most prevalent pathogen found in clinical mastitis cases in Canada.[8]

Classic short-duration antibiotic therapy against *S aureus* IMI is often unrewarding because of low cure rates during lactation.[7,9–13] New treatment regimens, such as extended therapy or combination of local and systemic antibiotic therapy, have been studied in the past decade to try to improve those cure rates.[7,11,14–19] Cure rate improvements observed in some of these studies have stimulated the interest of producers and veterinarians in those treatment regimens.

However, the studies were performed in many different countries, on different breeds, with different management practices and using several different antibiotics and dosage protocols against subclinical or clinical *S aureus* IMI. Consequently, comparison between studies should be made with caution.

The authors have nothing to disclose.

[a] Département des Sciences Cliniques, Faculté de Médecine Vétérinaire, 3200 rue Sicotte, CP 5000, St-Hyacinthe, Université de Montréal, Québec, Canada J2S 7C6.
[b] Department of Health Management, Atlantic Veterinary College, University of Prince Edward Island, 550 University Avenue, Charlottetown, Prince Edward Island, Canada C1A 4P3
* Corresponding author. 3200 rue Sicotte, CP 5000, St-Hyacinthe, Québec, Canada J2S 7C6.
E-mail address: jean-philippe.roy@umontreal.ca

doi:10.1016/j.cvfa.2011.12.004 vetfood.theclinics.com

Evidence-based medicine aims to apply the best available evidence gained from the scientific method to clinical decision making. Systematic reviews aim to identify, evaluate, and summarize the findings of all relevant individual studies, thereby making the available evidence more accessible to decision makers.[20] There is no systematic review available to help veterinarians choose the best lactational antibiotic therapy against *S aureus* IMI.

The objective of this report was therefore to perform a systematic review to answer the following clinical question: What is the best antibiotic treatment for *S aureus* IMI of lactating dairy cows in North America?

MATERIAL AND METHODS

Search Strategy

To answer the question, the following keywords were used by the authors: *Staph aureus* or *Staphylococcus aureus*; antibiotic(s) or antimicrobial(s); treatment or therapy; mastitis or intramammary infection or intra-mammary infection; bovine or cow(s) or cattle or milking cow(s) or dairy cow(s) or heifer(s). The equation used in all databases was: [(bovine or cow(s) or cattle or milking cow(s) or dairy cow(s) or heifer(s)) and (mastitis or intramammary infection or intra-mammary infection) and (*Staph aureus* or *Staphylococcus aureus*) and (antibiotic(s) or antimicrobial(s))] or [(bovine or cow(s) or cattle or milking cow(s) or dairy cow(s) or heifer(s)) and (mastitis or intramammary infection or intra-mammary infection) and (*Staph aureus* or *Staphylococcus aureus*) and (treatment or therapy)].

The initial web search was conducted by only one of the authors (JPR) in CAB database (1973–2011 week 32), PubMed database, and MEDLINE database (1948–2011 August week 1). No restriction was applied. Those databases were accessed August 17, 2011.

Identification of Relevant Studies

For each database, all titles were examined by one author (JPR). If the title was clearly unrelated to the clinical question, the article was excluded for further exploration. Then, for all titles that could be related to the question, abstracts were read by the same person. Reasons for exclusions at that step were as follows: study unrelated to the clinical question (including antibiotics not available in North America), abstract not available, article not written in English, and article not published in a peer-reviewed journal. Finally, the remaining articles were read by both authors. Some articles were still excluded at this last step because they did not involve the use of antibiotics available in North America or because there were no data from an original research project included in the articles. Those late exclusions were necessary because it was not possible to do it earlier in the process since some important data were not mentioned in the title or the abstract. Flow charts were used to report the selection and exclusion process.

Antibiotics available in North America to the authors knowledge are (1) lactating intramammary antibiotics: pirlimycin hydrochloride, cephapirin sodium, cloxacillin sodium, amoxicillin trihydrate, hetacillin potassium, penicillin G procaine, ceftiofur hydrochloride, and erythromycin; (2) systemic lactating cow antibiotics: oxytetracycline hydrochloride, penicillin G sodium, penicillin G procaine, ceftiofur hydrochloride or sodium, erythromycin, trimethoprim-sulfadoxine combination, sulfadimethoxine, and ampicillin trihydrate; and (3) nonlactating cow antibiotics: florfenicol, tulathromycin, tylosin, tilmicosin, and enrofloxacin. Not all systemic lactating cow antibiotics are labeled to treat mastitis but as labels varies among countries, readers should validate this issue with their country regulators. Another product, only available in Canada, is a combination of penicillin procaine, dihydrostreptomycin sulfate, novobiocin sodium, polymyxin B sulfate, hydrocortisone acetate, and hydrocortisone sodium succinate. No study was found using that specific formulation.

Selected Studies Assessment and Scoring

The remaining articles were assessed independently by both authors using the 100-point scaled version of the CONSORT 2010 checklist of information to include when reporting a randomized clinical trial (see article by Vandeweerd and colleagues elsewhere in this issue for further exploration of this topic). No attempt was made to obtain more details on any study by contacting researchers. A minimum score of 50 was used as the cut-off for inclusion. For articles with discordant results, the authors conducted a meeting to determine where scoring patterns diverged and to obtain a consensus.

Useful data on each article were recorded: authors, journal, year of publication, and country where the trial was performed. Data extracted on the methodology included randomization, blinding, treatment regimen, population studied, and group size. Outcome parameters studied were bacteriologic cure rates, new IMI rates, and post-treatment clinical mastitis incidence. Potential conflict of interest such as pharmaceutical company involvement as a funding source for the study or employer of at least one of the author was also recorded.

RESULTS

Figs. 1–3 shows flow charts of the study selection process. Briefly, 3082 titles were screened from the 3 databases. A total of 2889 titles were clearly unrelated to the clinical question and were excluded for further exploration. For the 193 titles that could be related to the question, 133 were excluded because of lack of relevance after abstract revision or because they were duplicates between database. An additional 40 articles were excluded because they were not published in English. Finally, the remaining articles (n = 20) were read by both authors.

Seven articles were excluded by the reviewers at this stage because they did not use antibiotics available in North America (n = 5) or because there were no data from an original research project included in the article (n = 2).

Of the remaining 13 articles, 5 articles were scored above 50 points by both reviewers for their quality and 5 articles were scored below 50 points. For the 3 articles with discordant results, consensus was reached after a discussion between the reviewers. As a result, 1 of the 3 articles was reclassified as meeting the criteria and the other 2 remained below the threshold. In total, 6 articles were included in the review.[9,14–16,19,21]

Table 1 summarizes the 6 articles that were retained. Five articles were randomized clinical trials with either a positive (treated) or negative (untreated) control. The sixth study was a large retrospective study, where cows were treated based on producer and veterinary treatment preference. In the retrospective study, treatment results were described for 7 antibiotics; however, only 4 antibiotics were used on more than 20 *S aureus* cases. Data for these antibiotic treatments are presented. Herds in all studies were commercial dairy herds with the exception of the study of Oliver and colleagues,[16] which used 3 University research herds. For Jarp and colleagues,[19] herd numbers were not specified, however, cases were recruited by 38 veterinary practitioners across 15 districts in Norway. For the retrospective study of Wilson and colleagues,[21] herd numbers were not specified; however, a very large number of screened samples from routine herd monitoring or high SCC investigations were included.

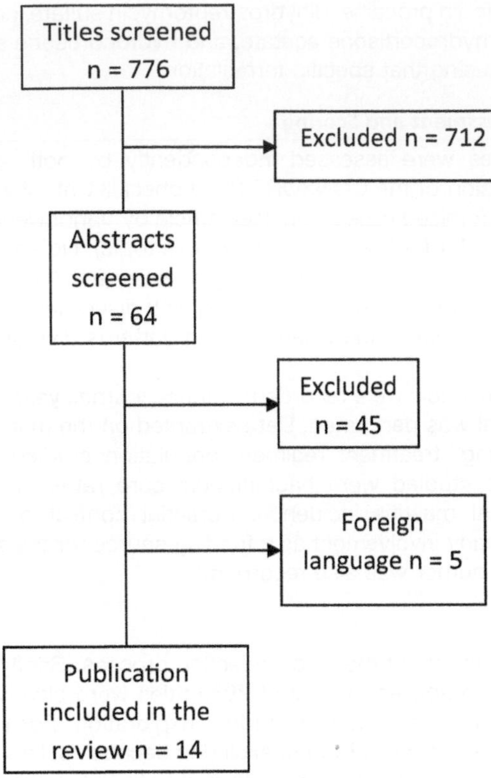

Fig. 1. Flow chart of selection process using PubMed database.

Recruitment practices and definitions of *S aureus* infection status at entry into the trial and definitions for cure of infection were different for each study. Some studies used milk culture–based diagnosis alone, while others used a combination of culture and SCC. The basic definitions are presented in **Table 2**. Four studies used subclinically infected cows only, 1 study used both subclinical and clinical cases, and 1 study used only clinically affected cows.

Definition of "infection cure" varied among the studies. Roy and colleagues[14] used the most restrictive definition for cure, requiring 3 negative follow-up cultures. Wilson and colleagues[9] required 3 negative cultures or 2 negative cultures and a low SCC. Oliver and colleagues[16] and Deluyker and colleagues[15] required 2 negative cultures to confirm cure, while Jarp and colleagues[19] and Wilson and colleagues[21] had only a single follow-up culture.

Results of treatment efficacy are presented in **Table 3**. Roy and colleagues[14] defined "cure" at both the quarter and cow level; however, full follow-up data were available only at the cow level because when a single quarter was found to be infected within the udder, sampling was discontinued for the entire cow. Conversely, for other studies cow level data were not presented. In the study of Roy and colleagues,[14] cow cure rate was higher (36.8%) for cows with one quarter infected versus 8.3% for cows with more than one quarter infected.

In general, cure rates for *S aureus* were low (<50%), with the exception of Deluyker and colleagues[15] and Wilson and colleagues.[22] Four of 6 studies showed significant

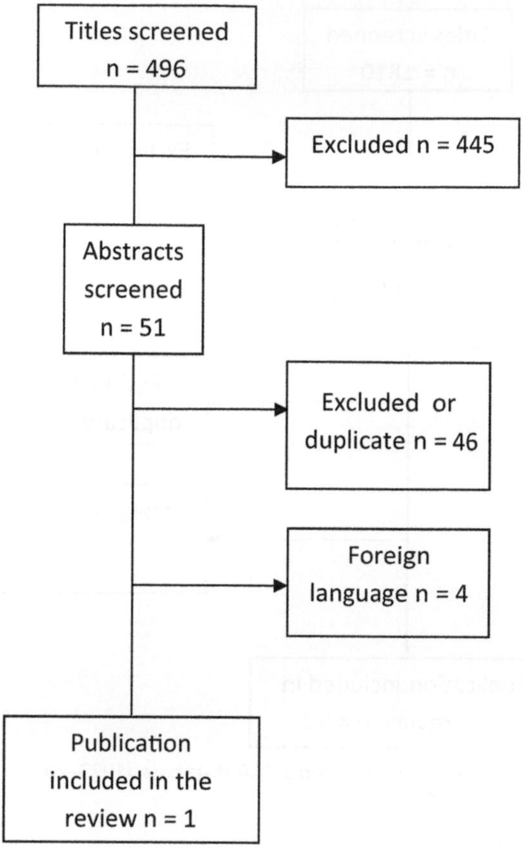

Fig. 2. Flow chart of selection process using MEDLINE database (1948–2011 August week 1).

treatment effects. Where duration of therapy with the same product was assessed (Deluyker and colleagues[15] and Oliver and colleagues[16]), longer-duration therapy had a positive association with cure rate. Only Jarp and colleagues[19] examined the impact of systemic versus systemic and intramammary therapy and, in fact, the product used for systemic therapy was different than the systemic/intramammary combination treatment. In that study, combination systemic/intramammary therapy with a combination penicillin/dihydrostreptomycin product was superior to 3 days of systemic therapy with penicillin and equivalent to 5 days of penicillin systemic treatment.

Clinical mastitis after extended therapy was reported in 2 studies (Roy and colleagues[14] and Deluyker and colleagues[15]). Roy and colleagues reported 4 cases (12.9%) of clinical mastitis of 31 cows treated. All cases were due to yeast IMI approximately 1 week after the end of the therapy. The authors in this study used sodium cephapirin 2 times a day for 5 days. Deluyker and colleagues reported an incidence of 5.2% of clinical mastitis in the group treated for 8 days with pirlimycin compared to 1.8% for the control group (pirlimycin for 2 days). These findings were also reported in other studies not keep in this systematic review[17,22] and constitute a potential drawback of extended therapy. Cow death following clinical mastitis after extended therapy using pirlimycin had been previously reported[17,22] but not in articles included in this systematic review.

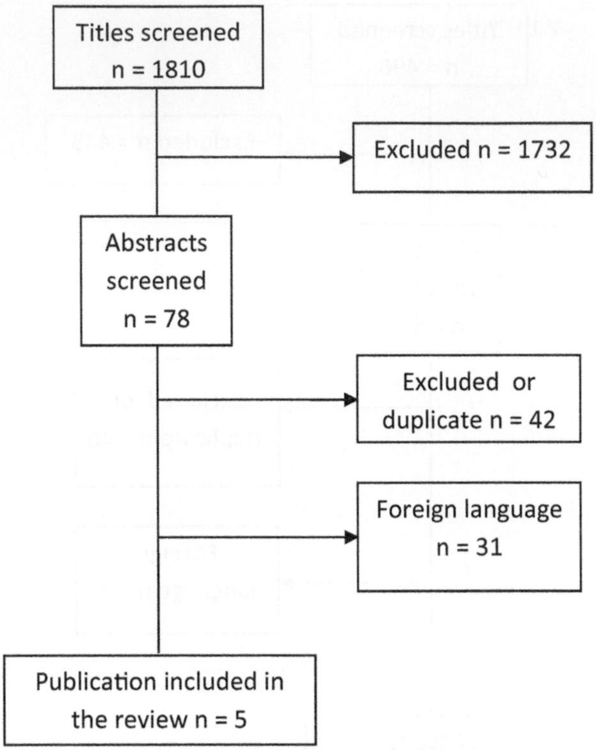

Fig. 3. Flow chart of selection process using CAB database (1973–2011 week 32).

In addition to treatment, Deluyker and colleagues[15] pretreatment SCC and quarter location (front vs back) were significantly associated with treatment response and older parity groups tended to have lower response to treatment.

DISCUSSION

This was the first time for both reviewers to conduct a systematic review using a scoring system. The authors are convinced that the process will increase validity of clinical decision-making and give a sound answer to the question asked.

However, some limitations on the process used should be reiterated before going further. Exclusion of publications was based on a rigorous application of the CONSORT 2010 checklist. Very few studies met the minimum criteria. No attempt was made to contact authors to add missing data to the published studies. Additionally, non–peer-reviewed publications were de facto excluded, as well as all non-English publications. Those decisions were made by the authors but could have been managed in a different way by others.

The 100-point scored version of the CONSORT 2010 checklist was used, (see article by Vandeweerd and colleagues elsewhere in this issue for further exploration of this topic) with a cut-off level for inclusion in the systematic review of 50 points. Consensus was apparent on 10 of 13 articles after initial review and agreement was reached on the final 3 articles after discussion between the authors. The majority of the articles lost points in several categories related to the material and methods

Table 1
Summary of study design features of 6 articles describing treatment efficacy during lactation against *S aureus* that met minimum selection criteria for inclusion in the systematic review

Author	Study Design	Number of Herds	*S aureus* Cases (n)	Treatment	Treatment Type	Controls
Roy et al[14]	Randomized clinical trial	14	61	Cephapirin sodium	5-day intramammary	Untreated
Deluyker et al[15]	Randomized clinical trial	54 (Study 1) 51 (Study 2)	140 122	Pirlimycin Pirlimycin	2-day intramammary 8-day intramammary	Untreated 2-day intramammary
Oliver et al[16]	Randomized clinical trial	3	50	Ceftiofur	2-, 5-, or 8-day intramammary	Untreated
Wilson et al[21]	Retrospective study[a]	Not specified	1272	Amoxicillin Cloxacillin Erythromycin Penicillin	Not described	Untreated
Wilson et al[9]	Randomized clinical trial	10	54	Florfenicol	3 intramammary treatments 12 hours apart	3 intramammary cloxacillin treatments 12 hours apart
Jarp et al[19]	Randomized clinical trial	Not specified	460	Penicillin	3 or 5 daily intramuscular treatments	1 intramuscular treatment of penicillin/dihydrostreptomycin followed by 4 daily intramammary treatments with a penicillin/ dihydrostreptomycin ointment

[a] Only antibiotic treatments with $\geq$20 cases are presented.

Table 2
Case definitions for enrolment and cure assessment for treatment efficacy against *S aureus*

Author	Case Definition	Cure Definition
Roy et al[14]	All cases subclinical Eligible if previous history of *S aureus* culture Enrolled if positive quarter culture on a minimum of 1 of 2 samples taken at 28 and 14 days prior to treatment	1. At quarter level, if *S aureus* was not recovered from previously infected quarters at 10, 24, and 31 days post treatment 2. At cow level, if all quarters were *S aureus* negative at 10, 24, and 31 days post treatment
Deluyker et al[15]	All cases subclinical Eligible if history of 2 consecutive SCC >250,000 or 1 >400,000 Enrolled if positive quarter culture and SCC >300,000 within 8 days of treatment	Negative for the pretreatment pathogen on quarter culture at 22–23 and 29–30 days post treatment
Oliver et al[16]	All cases subclinical Eligible if history of SCC >400,000 Enrolled if positive quarter culture on both of 2 samples taken 14 and 7 days prior to treatment	Negative for the pretreatment pathogen on quarter culture at 14 and 28 days post treatment
Wilson et al[21]	All cases subclinical Enrolled if positive quarter culture herd screening for which a second sample was recultured within 1 month	Negative for the pathogen identified by quarter herd screening on the subsequent sample taken within 1 month
Wilson et al[9]	**Subclinical cases** Eligible is previous history of *S aureus* culture Enrolled if positive quarter culture at time of enrollment **Clinical cases** Enrolled if bacterial pathogen present on both duplicate pretreatment milk samples from a cow with abnormal milk that did not have concurrent systemic signs	Same both subclinical and clinical Negative on quarter milk culture at days 14, 21, and 28 or negative on a minimum of 2 of these 3 samples with a SCC <300,000 on day 28
Jarp et al[19]	All cases clinical and subclinical cases coming from the same cows Cows in lactation 1, 2, or 3 and <6 months in lactation with abnormal secretion and/or visible signs of inflammation from which a penicillin-sensitive bacterium was cultured or quarters with no bacteria found but an increased SCC	Bacteriologic negative at 24–26 days and with low SCC for a quarter that had high SCC or a pathogen isolated on initial culture

Table 3
Summary of cure rates for treatment efficacy against *S aureus*

Author	Treatment	Cure Rate (n)	
		Subclinical	Clinical
Roy et al[14]	Negative control	3.3%[a] (1/30 cows)	NA
	5-day Intramammary Cephapirin sodium	25.8%[b] (8/31 cows)	NA
Deluyker et al[15]	Negative control	6 %[a] (4/63 quarters)[d]	NA
	2-day Intramammary Pirlimycin	56%[b] (82/146 quarters)[d]	NA
	8-day Intramammary Pirlimycin	86%[c] (46/53 quarters)[d]	NA
Oliver et al[16]	Negative control	0%[a] (0/12 quarters)	NA
	2-day ceftiofur	7%[a] (1/15 quarters)	
	5-day ceftiofur	17%[a,b] (2/12 quarters)	
	8-day ceftiofur	36%[b] (4/11 quarters)	
Wilson et al[21]	No treatment	43%[a] (471/1088 quarters)	NA
	Amoxicillin	43%[a] (30/70 quarters)	
Wilson et al[9]	Cloxacillin	47%[a] (23/49 quarters)	
	Erythromycin	65%[a] (15/23 quarters)	
	Penicillin	65%[a] (15/23 quarters)	17%[a] (2/12 quarters)
	Cloxacillin	6%[a] (1/17 quarters)	
	Florfenicol	0%[a] (0/14 quarters)	18%[a] (2/11 quarters)
Jarp et al[19]	Intramuscular penicillin/dihydrostreptomycin plus 4-day intramammary penicillin/dihydrostreptomycin	NA	40.6%[a] (54/133 quarters)
	3-day intramuscular penicillin		27.3%[b] (30/110 quarters)
	5-day intramuscular penicillin		46.8%[a] (59/126 quarters)

[a,b,c] Values within the same study with different superscripts are different ($P < .05$).
[d] Estimated based on models and sample size.

section, such as allocation ratio not presented, ethical protocol reference not presented, determination of the sample size not presented, and missing details about the random allocation (eg, methods used, by whom). Some points were also lost in other categories such as the introduction (eg, identification of a randomized trial in the title, presentation of the null hypothesis), the results section (eg, baseline demographic and clinical characteristics of each group, estimated effect size, and its precision), and the discussion (eg, trial limitations and source of potential bias, external validity), and the acknowledgment for the funding source of the research project was often not mentioned. Future articles should report more thoroughly the specific points just mentioned to allow a better comparison between studies. Researchers, reviewers, and editors should increase awareness of everyone involved in the process and make this issue a priority. Recently, guidelines to report trials and observational studies were published in veterinary journals.[23,24]

Direct comparison between studies has to be done with caution because of the large variation in study designs observed. One major variation observed is IMI and cure definitions. It is well established that milk bacteriology is not 100% sensitive. Dohoo and colleagues recently published a study that could be used to standardize these IMI definitions.[25] These definitions should be used in the future by researchers to report their work. That being said, some findings of this systematic review are valuable to discuss.

There is no evidence supporting combining systemic and local therapy for the control of *S. aureus* IMI during lactation. Only 1 study using that kind of approach was included in our systematic review.[19] More well-structured and -reported studies are needed in the future to evaluate this treatment regimen.

In general, cure rates for *S aureus* were low (<50%), with the exception of the rates of Deluyker and colleagues[15] and Wilson and colleagues.[21] Antibiotics used in those studies achieving higher cure rates were pirlimycin[15] and erythromycin or penicillin.[21] However, the latter study was a retrospective study and cure was assessed by only one milk culture approximately 30 days after clinical mastitis. Consequently, many factors could bias those results so they are less reliable. Considering this, pirlimycin seems to have the best cure rates among intramammary antibiotics. However, no direct comparison between antibiotics including pirlimycin is available so a definitive conclusion is impossible to make. Only Roy and colleagues reported cure rates at the cow level.[14] Decisions to attempt treatment versus cull for *S aureus* mastitis would typically be made at the cow rather than quarter level. Cure rates are inherently higher at the quarter level. Caution should be taken when extrapolating quarter level data to the cow-level decision.

Where duration of therapy with the same product was assessed, longer-duration therapy had a positive association with cure rate. This was done for pirlimycin[15] and ceftiofur.[16] Since all intramammary antibiotics are time-dependent antibiotics, it is logical that the longer the duration of the therapy, the better will be the results. Some drawbacks, like increased risk for clinical mastitis and treatment costs, should be considered and discussed with the producer before implementing such a treatment regimen.

The scope of this review was limited to antibiotic therapy. Cure rates for treatment depend on a number of cow and pathogen factors in addition to the therapeutic protocol. Cow factors include age, historical somatic cell count, duration of infection, and number of quarters infected. Pathogen factors include the numbers of colonies recoverable by culture and penicillin resistance. A full review of these risk factors was presented by Barkema and colleagues.[7]

SUMMARY

Based on this systematic review and considering available data, the best therapeutical option currently available in North America to treat *S aureus* IMI during lactation is an extended intramammary therapy for 5 to 8 days. Regarding specific antimicrobials, because direct comparison was not made among antibiotics and both enrollment and cure criteria at the cow and quarter level were inconsistent across studies, definitive conclusions are difficult. Pirlimycin seems to have higher cure rates at the quarter level than other studies reporting similar data and is labeled for extended therapy in both the United States and Canada. Caution should be exercised because several studies reported a spike in clinical mastitis rates following extended therapy. There is no evidence that a systemic antibiotic treatment should be combined to increase cure rates. More research is needed to validate those findings. Improvement is needed in research protocols including definition of IMI and cure and the publication process to facilitate evaluation and comparison between studies.

REFERENCES

1. Olde Riekerink RG, Barkema HW, Scholl DT, et al. Management practices associated with the bulk-milk prevalence of *Staphylococcus aureus* in Canadian dairy farms. Prev Vet Med 2010;97:20–8.
2. Petrovski KR, Heuer C, Parkinson TJ, et al. The incidence and aetiology of clinical bovine mastitis on 14 farms in Northland, New Zealand. N Z Vet J 2009;57:109–15.
3. Tenhagen BA, Hansen I, Reinecke A, et al. Prevalence of pathogens in milk samples of dairy cows with clinical mastitis and in heifers at first parturition. J Dairy Res 2009;76:179–87.
4. Ferguson JD, Azzaro G, Gambina M, et al. Prevalence of mastitis pathogens in Ragusa, Sicily, from 2000 to 2006. J Dairy Sci 2007;90:5798–813.
5. Piepers S, De Meulemeester L, de Kruif A, et al. Prevalence and distribution of mastitis pathogens in subclinically infected dairy cows in Flanders, Belgium. J Dairy Res 2007;74:478–83.
6. Osterås O, Sølverød L, Reksen O. Milk culture results in a large Norwegian survey: effects of season, parity, days in milk, resistance, and clustering. J Dairy Sci 2006;89:1010–23.
7. Barkema HW, Schukken YH, Zadoks RN. Invited review: The role of cow, pathogen, and treatment regimen in the therapeutic success of bovine *Staphylococcus aureus* mastitis. J Dairy Sci 2006;89:1877–95.
8. Olde Riekerink RG, Barkema HW, Kelton DF, et al. Incidence rate of clinical mastitis on Canadian dairy farms. J Dairy Sci 2008;91:1366–77.
9. Wilson DJ, Sears PM, Gonzalez RN, et al. Efficacy of florfenicol for treatment of clinical and subclinical bovine mastitis. AJVR 1996;57:526–8.
10. Owens WE, Nickerson SC, Ray CH. Efficacy of parenterally or intramammarily administered tilmicosin or ceftiofur against *Staphylococcus aureus* mastitis during lactation. J Dairy Sci 1999;82:645–7.
11. Owens WE, Ray CH, Boddie RL, et al. Efficacy of sequential intramammary antibiotic treatment against chronic *S. aureus* intramammary infection. Large Anim Pract 1997;Sep/Oct:10–4.
12. Sol J, Sampimon OC, Barkema HW, et al. Factors associated with cure after therapy of clinical mastitis caused by *Staphylococcus aureus*. J Dairy Sci 2000;83:278–84.
13. Owens WE, Watts JL, Boddie RL, et al. Antibiotic treatment of mastitis: comparison of intramammary and intramammary plus intramuscular therapies. J Dairy Sci 1988;71:3143–7.

14. Roy J-P, DesCôteaux L, DuTremblay D, et al. Efficacy of a 5-day extended therapy program during lactation with cephapirin sodium in dairy cows chronically infected with *Staphylococcus aureus*. Can Vet J 2009;50:1257–62.
15. Deluyker HA, Van Oye SN, Boucher JF. Factors affecting cure and somatic cell count after pirlimycin treatment of subclinical mastitis in lactating cows. J Dairy Sci 2005; 88:604–14.
16. Oliver SP, Gillepsie BE, Headrick SJ, et al. Efficacy of extended ceftiofur intramammary therapy for treatment of subclinical mastitis in lactating dairy cows. J Dairy Sci 2004;87:2393–400.
17. Gillespie BE, Moorehead H, Lunn P, et al. Efficacy of extended pirlimycin hydrochloride therapy for treatment of environmental *Streptococcus* spp and *Staphylococcus aureus* intramammary infections in lactating dairy cows. Vet Ther 2002;3:373–80.
18. Taponen S, Jantunen A, Pyorala E, et al. Efficacy of targeted 5-day combined parenteral and intramammary treatment of clinical mastitis caused by penicillin-susceptible or penicillin-resistant *Staphylococcus aureus*. Acta Vet Scand 2003;44: 53–62.
19. Jarp J, Bugge HP, Larsen S. Clinical trial of three therapeutic regimens for bovine mastitis. Vet Rec 1989;124:630–4.
20. Centre for Reviews and Dissemination. Systematic reviews: CRD's guidance for undertaking reviews in health care. York (UK): University of York; 2009.
21. Wilson DJ, Gonzalez RN, Case KL, et al. Comparison of seven antibiotic treatments with no treatment for bacteriological efficacy against bovine mastitis pathogens. J Dairy Sci 1999;82:1664–70.
22. Middleton JR, Luby CD. Escherichia coli mastitis in cattle being treated for Staphylococcus aureus intramammary infection. Vet Rec 2008;162:156–7.
23. O'Connor AM. Reporting guidelines for primary research: saying what you did. Prev Vet Med 2010;97:144–9.
24. Sargeant JM, O'Connor AM, Gardner IA, et al. The REFLECT statement: reporting guidelines for randomized controlled trials in livestock and food safety: explanation and elaboration. Food Prot 2010;73:579–603.
25. Dohoo IR, Smith J, Andersen S, et al. Diagnosis intramammary infection: evaluation of definitions based on a single milk sample. J Dairy Sci 2010;94:250–61.

Evidence-Based Use of Prokinetic Drugs for Abomasal Disorders in Cattle

Peter D. Constable, BVSc(Hons), MS, PhD[a,*],
Mohammad Nouri, DVM, PhD[b], Ismail Sen, DVM, PhD[c],
Aubrey N. Baird, MS, DVM[a], Thomas Wittek, Dr. habil[d]

KEYWORDS

- Macrolide • Erythromycin • Abomasum • Prokinetic
- Hypomotility

Impaired abomasal motility is common in dairy cattle and is suspected to play a major role in the development of left displaced abomasum (LDA), abomasal volvulus (AV), and abomasal impaction in adult cattle, and abomasal tympany in calves.[1,2] Abomasal emptying rate is decreased in cows with left displaced abomasum[3–5] and abomasal volvulus[4,6] and is further decreased immediately after surgical correction of left displaced abomasum.[4] A number of factors such as hypocalcemia,[7–9] endotoxemia,[10–12] alkalemia,[13,14] hyperglycemia and hyperinsulinemia,[15,16] and increased abomasal luminal osmolality and energy content[17–19] have been demonstrated to decrease abomasal emptying rate in adult cattle or milk-fed calves. Interestingly, fasting for 48 hours did not alter contractility of the pyloric antrum in adult cattle,[20] suggesting that short-term inappetance does not directly impact abomasal motility. Smooth muscle harvested from cattle with left displaced abomasum, right displaced

---

Research conducted by the authors that is the primary subject of discussion in the article has been supported, in part, by the Max Kade Foundation (New York), the United States Department of Agriculture Hatch Grant ILLU-70-0360, and BayerHealthCare AG, Germany.
Dr Constable has consultancy agreements with Boehringer-Ingelheim and Bayer Animal Health.
The authors have nothing to disclose.

[a] Department of Veterinary Clinical Sciences, Purdue University, 625 Harrison Street, West Lafayette, IN 47905-2026, USA
[b] Department of Clinical Sciences, College of Veterinary Medicine, Shahid Chamran University, Ahvaz, Iran
[c] Department of Internal Medicine, Faculty of Veterinary Medicine, University of Selcuk, Konya, Turkey
[d] Department for Farm Animals and Veterinary Public Health, University of Veterinary Medicine Vienna, Vienna, Austria
* Corresponding author.
E-mail address: constabl@purdue.edu

Vet Clin Food Anim 28 (2012) 51–70
doi:10.1016/j.cvfa.2011.12.008
vetfood.theclinics.com

abomasum, or abomasal volvulus exhibits a marked reduction in in vitro contractility,[21,22] indicating that abomasal hypomotility should be assumed to be present in all cattle with abomasal displacement and volvulus. It would therefore be clinically helpful to identify effective therapeutic agents that stimulate, coordinate, and restore abomasal motility in cattle. Such therapeutic agents are termed prokinetics.[23]

Abomasal emptying in adult ruminants and milk-fed calves is best characterized as fluid emptying, rather than semisolid or solid emptying.[24,25] It is widely accepted that the rate of gastric (and therefore abomasal) fluid emptying is determined by the interaction between the tone of the gastric body, antral contractility, pyloric resistance, duodenal resistance, and gastroduodenal coordination, with the pressure gradient between the stomach and duodenum being the most important determinant of emptying rate after ingesting a fluid meal.[26,27] For comparison, the rate of gastric emptying after ingestion of a solid meal is controlled largely by antral contractions.[26] After ingestion of a fluid meal, the pressure gradient between the stomach and duodenum is created by rapid phasic contractions of the gastric body superimposed on slower sustained contractions, and the rate of liquid emptying increases linearly with luminal pressure.[26]

Acetylcholine, norepinephrine (noradrenaline), and epinephrine (adrenaline) are the most important neurotransmitters in the ruminant autonomic nervous system,[28] with acetylcholine acting through muscarinic acetylcholine receptors (M) and norepinephrine and epinephrine acting through different subtypes of α- and β-adrenergic receptors (ARs).[29] Opioid, dopaminergic, and serotonin receptors also appear to play a role in modulating gastrointestinal motility in ruminants, but their relative influence on abomasal motility appears to be much less than that of acetylcholine, norepinephrine, and epinephrine. The innervation pattern of the bovine abomasum is different from the gastric muscle layers in monogastric animals[28]; this observation suggests that effective prokinetic drugs in monogastric animals may not necessarily be effective in cattle.

Therapeutic options in the treatment of abomasal hypomotility have been the subject of previous reviews.[23,30] The main aim of this review was to identify and summarize the available evidence regarding drugs that could be effective prokinetic agents for cattle with abomasal hypomotility. The intent was to develop evidence-based recommendations for the treatment and prevention of abomasal hypomotility in cattle and to identify potentially valuable areas for future investigation.

METHODS

Electronic databases were searched using CAB Direct (1910 to present) and MEDLINE (PubMed 1965 to present). The initial search terms were abomasal OR abomasum AND motility OR hypomotility OR atony OR emptying AND cattle.

The CAB Direct search provided 765 citations and the MEDLINE search provided 290 citations. Titles and abstracts for all publications were read by the first author, and those that did not relate to abomasal motility in cattle, sheep, or goats were discarded. Bibliographies from retained publications were read and additional publications were identified. A search conducted using Google Scholar and similar initial search terms was also used to identify publications not indexed by CAB Direct and MEDLINE.

Meta-analyses or systematic reviews were not available. Emphasis in this review was therefore placed on the results from 5 clinical trials conducted on adult cattle with abomasal hypomotility due to left displaced abomasum[5,31–33] or abomasal volvulus.[6] Because the number of clinical trials was small, additional emphasis was placed on the results from 6 randomized controlled studies performed on healthy adult cattle[34,35] and milk-fed calves.[2,36–38] The findings of 7 in vitro studies using bovine abomasal tissue were also reviewed, although evidence obtained from these studies is not as strong and clinically applicable as the results from randomized controlled clinical trials. Treatments for abomasal hypomotility in cattle were categorized as proven effective (macrolides), potentially effective (parasympathomimetics, calcium, potassium), or proven ineffective (flunixin meglumine, metoclopramide). Categorization as proven effective was based on statistical significance in a controlled clinical trial in healthy or diseased cattle. Categorization as potentially effective was based on statistical significance in an in vitro study using bovine abomasal tissue. Categorization as proven ineffective was based on the absence of statistical significance in an appropriately powered and controlled clinical trial in healthy or diseased cattle.

PROVEN EFFECTIVE TREATMENTS FOR ABOMASAL HYPOMOTILITY

Macrolides

Macrolides are a group of closely related antimicrobials that are categorized according to the number of macrocyclic lactone ring components as 12-membered, 13-membered, 14-membered, 15-membered, and 16-membered groups, with one or more amino sugars or deoxy sugars being attached to the lactone ring. Erythromycin (14-membered), gamithromycin (15-membered), spiramycin (16-membered), tilmicosin (16-membered), tulathromycin (13- and 15-membered), and tylosin (16-membered) are currently approved and marketed for veterinary use, with availability varying from country to country. Macrolides have pharmacodynamic properties beyond their antimicrobial effects, including anti-inflammatory and immunomodulatory properties, that are perceived to be clinically beneficial.[39] Studies from our laboratories have demonstrated that an additional pharmacodynamic property of macrolides is a prokinetic effect.

The prokinetic effect of erythromycin is marked and consequently has been extensively investigated in humans and animals. Erythromycin induces phase III of the interdigestive migrating motor complex (MMC), increases the amplitude of antral contractions, and improves antroduodenal coordination in a number of species.[40,41] Erythromycin appears to exert its prokinetic effect primarily by acting as a motilin-receptor agonist via binding to motilin receptors in the pyloric antrum and proximal portion of the small intestine.[42] Motilin is a peptide consisting of 22 amino acids that is periodically released from endocrine cells in the duodenojejunal mucosa, thereby initiating the MMC of the mammalian gastrointestinal tract during the interdigestive period. There is considerable interest in the group of nonpeptide motilin agonists, referred to as the motilides (ie, motilin-like macrolides), that interact with the motilin receptor and promote gastric emptying.[42]

Structure-activity studies have indicated that motilides have 3 main structural requirements that enable them to interact strongly with the motilin receptor and thereby induce changes in gastrointestinal motility: a ring structure (typically a 14-member lactone ring), an amino sugar (desosamine) bound at C-5 of the ring in a glycosidic linkage, and a neutral sugar (such as cladinose) bound at C-3 of the ring in a glycosidic linkage.[43,44] From this 3-part structure, the potency of the motilide is influenced primarily by modifications to the N-dimethylamino group at the 3′ position of the amino sugar bound at C-5 of the ring and, to a lesser extent, the configuration of the lactone ring structure (C-6 through C-9) and by the presence of a neutral sugar at C-3 that is parallel to the amino sugar at C-5.[45] Accordingly, it is likely that the 6 macrolides currently approved and marketed for veterinary use (erythromycin, gamithromycin, spiramycin, tilmicosin, tulathromycin, and tylosin) will have variable prokinetic activity, with erythromycin having the most pronounced effect on promoting

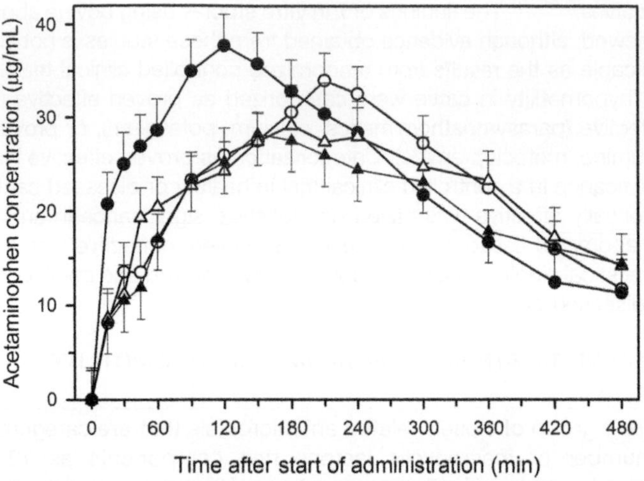

Fig. 1. Changes in plasma acetaminophen concentrations in 7 Holstein-Friesian calves. Values reported are least squares mean ± SE. Calves received each of 4 treatments in random order (2 mL of saline [0.9% NaCl] solution, IM [control treatment; white circles]; erythromycin, 8.8 mg/kg, IM [black circles]; tilmicosin, 10 mg/kg, SC [white triangles]; and tylosin, 17.6 mg/kg, IM [black triangles]). Calves were fed 2 L of milk replacer containing acetaminophen (50 mg/kg) 30 minutes later. Onset of suckling was designated as time 0. (*From* Nouri M, Constable PD. Effect of parenteral administration of erythromycin, tilmicosin, and tylosin on abomasal emptying rate in suckling calves. Am J Vet Res 2007;68:1392–8; with permission.)

abomasal motility. Studies have been conducted documenting the prokinetic effects of erythromycin, spiramycin, tilmicosin, tulathromycin, and tylosin in cattle.

Studies in milk-fed calves

The first randomized controlled cross-over study to demonstrate that erythromycin was an effective prokinetic agent when administered at the labeled antimicrobial dose was performed by Wittek and Constable and published in 2005.[2] Administration of erythromycin (8.8 mg/kg, IM) caused an immediate and profound increase in mean luminal pressure, abomasal motility and emptying rate in 6 healthy milk-fed calves. Interestingly, administration of erythromycin at 0.88 mg/kg IM in the same study did not have a detectable effect on mean luminal pressure and emptying rate.[2] The mechanism by which erythromycin increased abomasal emptying rate appeared to be related to an increased frequency of luminal pressure waves and increased mean luminal pressure, as well as increased antroduodenal coordination.[2]

In a follow-up randomized controlled study in 2007, Nouri and Constable investigated the effect of parenteral administration of erythromycin, tilmicosin, and tylosin administered at the label dose rate on abomasal emptying rate in 7 milk-fed Holstein-Friesian bull calves less than 35 days old.[36] Calves were administered each of 4 treatments in random order using a cross-over study design (2 mL of saline [0.9% NaCl] solution, IM [control treatment]; erythromycin, 8.8 mg/kg, IM; tilmicosin, 10 mg/kg, SC; and tylosin, 17.6 mg/kg, IM). Erythromycin, tilmicosin, and tylosin administration resulted in a faster rate of emptying than the control treatment as determined on the basis of time to pharmacokinetically determined maximal plasma acetaminophen concentration (**Fig. 1**). Ultrasonography indicated that the half-time of abomasal emptying was significantly shorter for erythromycin than for the control treatment. Tilmicosin and tylosin accelerated the abomasal emptying rate, but not significantly as assessed by ultrasonography, relative to the emptying rate for the control treatment.[36] This study confirmed the previous study[2] that erythromycin was an effective prokinetic agent in milk-fed calves, and suggested for the first time that two macrolides with a 16-membered lactone ring (tilmicosin, tylosin) had prokinetic activity when administered at the label dosage, albeit reduced compared to erythromycin.

The prokinetic effect of erythromycin in healthy milk-fed calves was also confirmed by Nouri and colleagues in 2008 in a randomized controlled study using a cross-over design.[37] Five Holstein-Friesian bull calves (8–15 days of age) received each of the following 4 IM treatments in random order: control, 2 mL of 0.9% NaCl; erythromycin, 8.8 mg/kg; low-dose gentamicin, 4.4 mg/kg; high-dose gentamicin, 6.6 mg/kg. Erythromycin increased abomasal emptying rate, as indicated by a shorter time to pharmacokinetically determined maximal plasma acetaminophen concentration, whereas low- and high-dose gentamicin administration did not change abomasal emptying rate.[37]

The effect of parenteral administration of erythromycin or ivermectin on the abomasal emptying rate was investigated in a randomized controlled study using 6 male Holstein-Friesian calves less than 15 days old.[38] Ivermectin is classified as a macrocyclic lactone but has a number of structural differences from erythromycin that are related to its antiparasitic activity. In a crossover study, calves were administered each of 3 treatments (erythromycin, 8.8 mg/kg, IM; ivermectin, 200 μg/kg, IV; control treatment, 2 mL of saline [0.9% NaCl] solution, IM). Calves were bottle fed 2 L of fresh cow's milk containing acetaminophen (50 mg/kg) 30 minutes later and blood samples were periodically collected from the jugular vein. Abomasal emptying rate was assessed by use of the time to pharmacokinetically determined maximal plasma acetaminophen concentration. Both erythromycin and ivermectin significantly increase the abomasal emptying rate, compared with results for the control treatment.[38] The clinical significance of a small increase in abomasal emptying rate after IV administration of ivermectin remains to be determined because ivermectin is only labeled for SC, oral, and topical administration.

Studies in adult cattle

In a preliminary study in lactating dairy cows, administration of erythromycin lactobionate at 2 doses (0.1 mg/kg, IV or 1 mg/kg, IV or IM) or erythromycin base (10 mg/kg, IM) in polyethylene glycol each resulted in a large and sustained increase in the myoelectrical activity in the abomasal body, pyloric antrum, and duodenum and an increase in the luminal pressure in the abomasal body, compared with untreated cattle.[35] These effects were accompanied by an increased rate of abomasal emptying, as assessed by change in duodenal pH.

The first clinical trial to investigate the effect of preoperative administration of erythromycin on postoperative abomasal emptying rate in dairy cows undergoing surgical correction of left displacement of the abomasum was conducted by Wittek and colleagues in 2008.[5] Forty-five lactating Holstein-Friesian cows with left displaced abomasum were alternately assigned to treatment with erythromycin (10 mg/kg, IM), the nonsteroidal anti-inflammatory agent flunixin meglumine (2.2 mg/kg, IV), or an untreated control group with 15 cows per group. Treatments were administered once 1 hour before surgical correction of left displaced abomasum by right flank omentopexy with the cow in a standing position. Abomasal emptying rate was determined by injecting D-xylose solution (50% solution; 0.5 g/kg) into the abomasal lumen during surgery and venous blood samples were periodically obtained

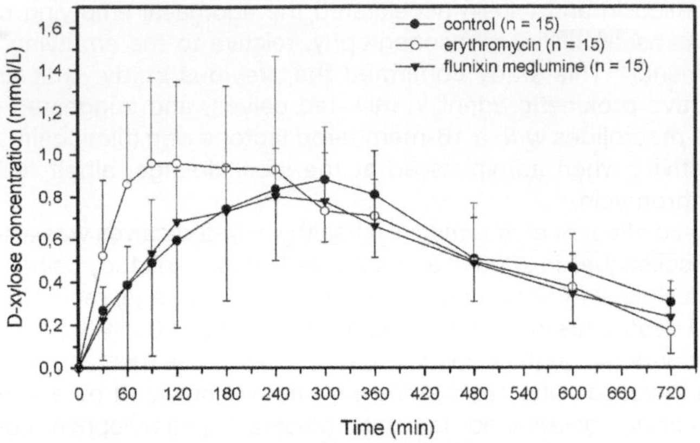

Fig. 2. Mean serum D-xylose concentration in 45 dairy cows undergoing surgical correction of LDA that were not given any specific treatments to prevent postoperative hypomotility of the gastrointestinal tract (control), were given a single dose of erythromycin (10 mg/kg [4.5 mg/lb], IM) 1 hour prior to surgery, or were given a single dose of flunixin meglumine (2.2 mg/kg [1.0 mg/lb], IV) 1 hour prior to surgery. A 50% solution of D-xylose (1 mL/kg [0.45 mL/lb]) was injected into the abomasal lumen at the time of surgery (time 0). Error bars represent SD. (*From* Wittek T, Tischer K, Gieseler T, et al. Effect of preoperative administration of erythromycin or flunixin meglumine on postoperative abomasal emptying rate in dairy cows undergoing surgical correction of left displacement of the abomasum. J Am Vet Med Assoc 2008;232:418–23; with permission.)

to determine the time to maximum serum D-xylose concentration. Abomasal emptying rate was significantly faster in cows treated with erythromycin than in control cows but was not significantly different between cows treated with flunixin meglumine and control cows (**Fig. 2**). Cows in the erythromycin- and flunixin meglumine–treated groups had a significantly higher rumen contraction rate on the first postoperative day than did control cows (**Fig. 3**).[5] Cows treated with erythromycin had significantly greater milk production, relative to production before surgery, on postoperative days 1 and 2 than did control cows (**Fig. 4**). The results indicated that preoperative administration of a single dose of erythromycin increased abomasal emptying rate, rumen contraction rate, and milk production in the immediate postoperative period in cows undergoing surgical correction of left displaced abomasum.

In a related clinical trial using a convenience sample, Wittek and colleagues investigated the effects of preoperative erythromycin or combined dexamethasone/vitamin C treatment on postoperative abomasal emptying rate in cows undergoing surgical correction of abomasal volvulus.[6] Forty-five lactating Holstein-Friesian cows with abomasal volvulus were alternately assigned to treatment with erythromycin (10 mg/kg body weight [BW], IM), the glucocorticoid anti-inflammatory agent dexamethasone (0.02 mg/kg BW, IV) combined with vitamin C (10 mg/kg BW, IV), or no treatment (control group) with 15 cows per group. Dexamethasone and vitamin C were coadministered in an attempt to investigate the efficacy of antioxidative agents in preventing reperfusion injury. Treatments were administered 1 hour before surgical correction of abomasal volvulus by right flank omentopexy with the cow in a standing position. Abomasal emptying rate was determined by injecting D-xylose solution (50% solution; 0.5 g/kg) into the abomasal lumen during surgery, and venous blood samples were periodically obtained to determine the time to maximum serum

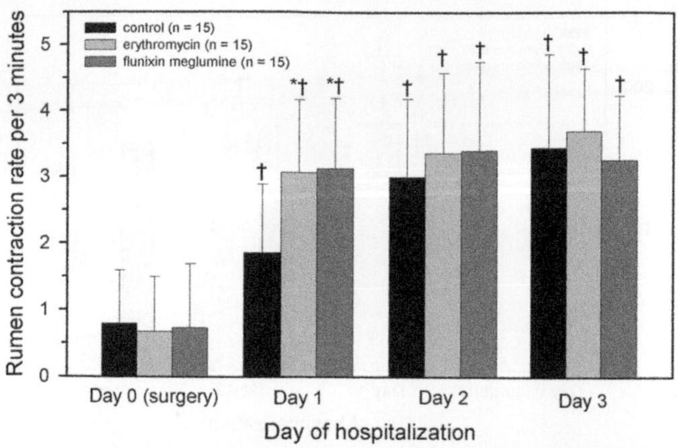

Fig. 3. Mean rumen contraction rate (ie, number of contractions in 3 minutes) for dairy cows undergoing surgical correction of LDA that were not given any specific treatments to prevent postoperative hypomotility of the gastrointestinal tract (control) or were given a single dose of erythromycin or flunixin meglumine. Error bars represent SD. *Significantly ($P<.05$) different from value for control group cows on the same day. †Significantly ($P<.005$) different from value obtained on day 0 for the same group. (*From* Wittek T, Tischer K, Gieseler T, et al. Effect of preoperative administration of erythromycin or flunixin meglumine on postoperative abomasal emptying rate in dairy cows undergoing surgical correction of left displacement of the abomasum. J Am Vet Med Assoc 2008;232:418–23; with permission.)

D-xylose concentration. Abomasal emptying rate was significantly faster in cows administered erythromycin than untreated controls, whereas abomasal emptying rate was similar in control cows and cows receiving dexamethasone and vitamin C (**Fig. 5**).[6] Both erythromycin and dexamethasone/vitamin C treatment improved postoperative milk yield within 1 day after surgery. The results indicated that preoperative injection of erythromycin (10 mg/kg BW, IM) is an effective method for ameliorating postoperative abomasal hypomotility in cows with abomasal volvulus. Because clinical signs of abomasal hypomotility are evident on day 2 to 5 after surgical correction of abomasal volvulus,[46] consideration should be given to daily treatment with erythromycin for the first 5 postoperative days.[30] This supposition needs to be verified with an appropriately designed randomized clinical trial.

Although yet to be investigated, it is likely that the prokinetic effect of macrolides remains after repeated administration in adult cattle and milk-fed calves. This is because a prokinetic effect was maintained in humans with diabetic gastroparesis after 4 weeks of oral administration of erythromycin,[47] and clinically relevant concentrations of erythromycin do not alter motilin receptor density in rabbits.[48]

Antimicrobials are commonly administered during the perioperative period when surgical correction of left displaced abomasum is performed on the farm, because surgery is often performed in a less-than-ideal environment and because many cattle with left displaced abomasum have concurrent diseases such as metritis, retained placenta, and mastitis.[1] Antimicrobials commonly administered to lactating dairy cattle in the perioperative period include procaine penicillin G, amoxicillin, ceftiofur, and oxytetracycline, with antimicrobials selected on the basis of treatment efficacy and milk withdrawal times.[2] The documented effects of erythromycin in promoting abomasal motility raises the interesting question as to whether erythromycin is the preferred antimicrobial for perioperative administration in cattle undergoing surgical correction of

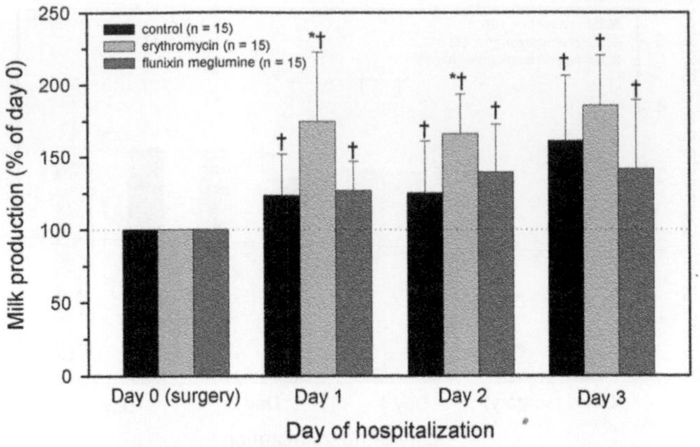

Fig. 4. Mean relative daily milk production (ie, milk production as a percentage of production on day 0) for dairy cows undergoing surgical correction of LDA that were not given any specific treatments to prevent postoperative hypomotility of the gastrointestinal tract (control) or were given a single dose of erythromycin or flunixin meglumine. Error bars represent SD. *Significantly ($P<.05$) different from value for control group cows on the same day. †Significantly ($P<.005$) different from baseline value (100%) for the same group. (*From* Wittek T, Tischer K, Gieseler T, et al. Effect of preoperative administration of erythromycin or flunixin meglumine on postoperative abomasal emptying rate in dairy cows undergoing surgical correction of left displacement of the abomasum. J Am Vet Med Assoc 2008;232:418–23; with permission.)

left displaced abomasum. However, studies are needed to compare the cost and efficacy of erythromycin with the cost and efficacy of antimicrobial agents such as procaine penicillin in the perioperative period in cattle with left displaced abomasum.

POTENTIALLY EFFECTIVE TREATMENTS FOR ABOMASAL HYPOMOTILITY

Parasympathomimetic Agents

The parasympathomimetic agents carbamylcholine, bethanechol, and neostigmine have been administered to cattle with left displaced abomasum, right displaced abomasum, and abomasal volvulus in an attempt to increase abomasal motility. Five subtypes (M_1–M_5) of the acetylcholine M receptor have been identified, and a marked site-specific distribution of the 5 M subtypes has been reported in cattle.[49] The M_2 and M_3 subtypes are by far the most abundant M receptors in cattle and are localized to different compartments of smooth muscle cells, with M_3 being located on the nerve terminals innervating smooth muscle cells.[50] Binding of an agonist to the more prevalent M_2 receptor inhibits adenylate cyclase activity, whereas binding of an agonist to M_3 activates phospholipase C.[51] The M_3 receptor subtype is considered to be the most important subtype in eliciting smooth muscle contraction in cattle.[22]

In general, parasympathetic nervous system activation increases gastrointestinal smooth muscle tone. This may, or may not, be accompanied by an increase in motility. Atropine is a nonselective blocker for all 5 M subtypes that induces atony of the reticulorumen[52] and abomasum[9] when administered at 0.04 mg/kg IV in cattle. In contrast, the direct acting parasympathomimetic agent bethanechol, which is a methyl derivative of carbamylcholine, increases smooth muscle contractility of abomasal antral and intestinal tissue of dairy cows by acting as a muscarinic acetylcholine receptor agonist primarily through M_3 and, to a lesser extent, through M_2 receptor

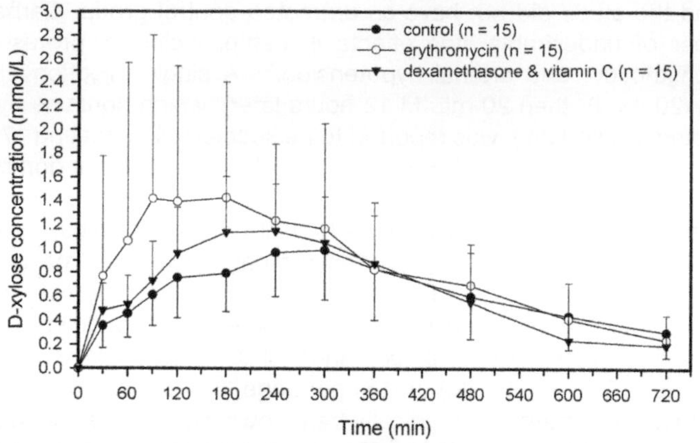

Fig. 5. Serum D-xylose concentration in lactating cows after surgical correction of abomasal volvulus. A D-xylose solution (50%, 0.5 g/kg body weight) was injected into the abomasal lumen during surgical correction at time = 0 min. Cows of group E (n = 15) were treated 1 hour before surgical correction with erythromycin (10 mg/kg IM), cows of group D (n = 15) were treated 1 hour before surgical correction with dexamethasone (0.02 mg/kg IV) and vitamin C (10 mg/kg IV). Cows of group C (n = 15) served as untreated control. Values are mean ± SD. (*From* Wittek T, Tischer K, Körner I, et al. Effect of preoperative erythromycin or dexamethasone/vitamin C on postoperative abomasal emptying rate in dairy cows undergoing surgical correction of abomasal volvulus. Vet Surg 2008;37:537–44; with permission.)

subtypes.[22,53–55] Bethanechol is more resistant to cholinesterase than acetylcholine and therefore has a longer duration of action than acetylcholine.[22] Bethanechol and carbamylcholine should be injected subcutaneously because intramuscular injection can result in localized skeletal muscle contraction. A subcutaneous dose rate of 0.07 mg/kg for bethanechol does not produce undesirable side effects in cattle.[23,34]

The results of in vitro studies have demonstrated that bethanechol induces a significant and concentration-dependent increase in contractility in smooth muscle from the fundus, corpus, and pyloric antrum of healthy cattle, with a more marked effect on contraction of the fundus and corpus.[54,56] Interestingly, bethanechol produced a greater increase in contractility of circular smooth muscle than longitudinal smooth muscle.[54] Two in vitro studies examining the contractility of abomasal tissue from cattle with displaced abomasum demonstrated a decreased responsiveness to acetylcholine[21] and bethanechol,[22] which was consistent with impaired intrinsic muscle motility. The results of recent in vitro studies indicated that the density of M_2 and M_3 receptors in the abomasum of cattle with LDA was similar to that of healthy control cows[29] but that there was a reduced responsiveness to bethanechol in the abomasum of cows with LDA.[22] Taken together, the results of these 3 in vitro studies suggest that parasympathomimetic agents may have some therapeutic value in treating abomasal hypomotility, particularly related to left displaced abomasum.

A single injection of carbamylcholine (6 mg, SC) was reported to be successful in treating 3 cows with left displaced abomasum.[57] However, this study was not randomized and did not have an untreated control group. Repeated injections of carbamylcholine (50 mg SC daily for 5 days) were reported to be successful in treating 26 of 29 cows with right displaced abomasum.[58] However, this study was not randomized, the criteria for a diagnosis of right displaced abomasum were not provided, and the study did not have an untreated control group. Carbamylcholine has a number of undesirable side effects in cattle, including profuse salivation, bronchial constriction, and arterial hypotension.[59] A single injection of Buscopan compositum (20 mL IV then 20 mL IM 12 hours later), which contains hyoscine and dipyrone (metamizol sodium), was reported to be successful in treating 17 of 22 cows with right displaced abomasum.[60] However, this study was not randomized and did not have an untreated control group, and a close inspection of the manuscript indicates that some of the enrolled cows had abomasal volvulus, which requires immediate surgical correction. The reported clinical "successes" of treatment with carbamylcholine (a parasympathomimetic) and hyoscine (a parasympatholytic similar to atropine) that have opposite activities cannot be easily reconciled.

Twice-daily oral administration of bethanechol (0.1 mg/kg) was combined with metoclopramide (0.2–1 mg/kg, IM) or domperidone (0.2–2.5 mg/kg, IM) and aspirin (100 mg/kg, PO) in an attempt to medically treat cows with left displaced abomasum, with a success rate of less than 50%.[3] This study was not randomized and did not have an untreated control group. In the only randomized crossover in vivo study conducted to date, SC administration of bethanechol (0.07 mg/kg) to healthy yearling cattle induced minor changes in electromyographic activity of the pyloric antrum that may reflect a prokinetic effect; however, the authors stated that myoelectrical activity does not always correlate with flow of digesta.[34]

Administration of the reversible acetylcholinesterase inhibitor neostigmine (0.012 mg/kg, IV) appeared to increase abomasal smooth muscle contractility in calves, as assessed by electromyography.[61] However, in milk-fed calves, neostigmine (0.04 mg/kg, IM) did not change the transit time to the ileum.[62] Moreover, in a randomized controlled cross-over study in healthy calves, neostigmine (0.02 mg/kg, SC twice 2 hours apart) did not alter abomasal motility, pressure, or emptying rate in milk-fed calves.[2] These 2 randomized controlled studies provide strong evidence that neostigmine does not increase abomasal emptying rate in milk-fed calves. Neostigmine may even be deleterious to abomasal emptying because coadministration of neostigmine (0.02 mg/kg, SC twice 2 hours apart) with erythromycin (8.8 mg/kg, IM once) partially ameliorated the prokinetic effect of erythromycin in healthy milk-fed calves.[2] A neostigmine-induced increase in pyloric or duodenal tone[63] provides a possible explanation for this finding.

Sympatholytic, Anti-Inflammatory, and Analgesic Agents

Receptors for norepinephrine and epinephrine are widely expressed in ruminant tissue, with marked site-specific distribution and abundance within the gastrointestinal tract of dairy cows.[64] Specifically, the α-AR subtype α_{2AD} and the β-AR subtype β_2 are the most abundant.[64] Investigations have demonstrated that the α_2-AR is located presynaptically on cholinergic axons, whereas the β_2-AR is located postsynaptically on gastrointestinal smooth muscle cells.[29] Stimulation of the α_2-AR results in inhibition of adenylate cyclase activity and decrease in cyclic adenosine monophosphate–dependent sequestration of intracellular calcium, thereby decreasing smooth muscle tone.[29] Stimulation of β_2-AR results in activation of adenylate cyclase activity and increases intracellular cAMP levels.[29]

Although the administration of α_2-AR agonists such as xylazine to cattle causes a dose-dependent inhibition of reticuloruminal motility,[52] xylazine has been demonstrated to be a transient prokinetic agent in cattle with experimentally induced abomasal hypomotility. Administration of xylazine (0.2 mg/kg, IM) to cattle 15 minutes after pretreatment with atropine (0.05 mg/kg, IM) produced an immediate, marked, and sustained increase in the contractile force of the pyloric antrum of 3 cows that lasted approximately 3 to 6 hours depending on the days of fasting.[20] The prokinetic effect on the pyloric antrum was associated with an inhibition of duodenal motility, and the combined effect on motility was assumed to promote abomasal emptying. The prokinetic effect on the abomasum is consistent with xylazine activation of the α_2-AR in circular smooth muscle in the pyloric antrum.[28] A similar increase in contractile activity of the pyloric antrum was reported in 4 dairy cows administered xylazine (0.2 mg/kg, IV) or medetomidine (0.01 mg/kg).[20] There is one report of an uncontrolled study where administration of α_2-agonists to sedate cattle with left displaced abomasum and subsequent rolling was successful in treating the displaced abomasum in 5 of 6 cows. The authors reported a marked increase in the intensity of sounds in the right flank of the cattle during auscultation immediately after rolling that was attributed to administration of the α_2-agonist.[20]

Electroacupuncture has been used as part of the treatment for left displaced abomasum, using daily stimulation of 3 acupoints for 3 consecutive days, with or without the administration of neostigmine (0.01 mg/kg SC) or application of a modified Moxa patch.[65] The treatment was reported to be effective in 9 of 12 cows; however, the study was not randomized and did not have an untreated control group.

Calcium if Hypocalcemia Is Present

It is axiomatic that smooth muscle contraction, including abomasal smooth muscle, is dependent, in part, on the calcium concentration in the cytosol. It is also axiomatic that cytosolic calcium concentration is dependent, in part, on plasma calcium concentration. The influence of hypocalcemia on abomasal emptying rate was first reported in 1974 with a study on goats with experimentally induced hypocalcemia.[13] This study led to recommendations that calcium administration was indicated as part of the treatment of left displaced abomasum.[8] Subsequent studies suggested that abomasal motility appears to be less sensitive to reductions in plasma ionized calcium concentration than does reticuloruminal motility in sheep[66] and presumably cattle. During experimentally induced hypocalcemia, a linear relationship exists between rumen contraction amplitude and serum ionized calcium concentration,[66] and it was assumed that a similar linear relationship existed between abomasal contraction amplitude and serum ionized calcium concentration. However, in a 1983 study, a curvilinear relationship was observed between both the number and amplitude of abomasal contractions and plasma total calcium concentration in 5 cattle with experimentally induced hypocalcemia,[7] with motility being markedly decreased when the total calcium concentration was less than 1.3 mmol/L. The results of a 1988 study in 2 cattle with experimentally induced hypocalcemia also indicated a marked decrease in abomasal motility occured when total calcium concentration was less than 1.2 mmol/L.[9] A 2003 study in 3 cows with experimentally induced hypocalcemia confirmed that reticuloruminal motility was more sensitive to decreased plasma calcium concentration than abomasal motility and that the pyloric antral region was more sensitive to hypocalcemia than the abomasal fundus.[67] Taken together, the results of 5 in vivo studies in healthy cattle, sheep, and goats with experimentally induced hypocalcemia indicate that marked hypocalcemia can decrease abomasal hypomotility but that the effect of mild hypocalcemia on abomasal motility remains to be determined.

Two observational studies showed no association between subclinical hypocalcemia and subsequent development of left displaced abomasum in dairy cattle.[68,69] In contrast, an often-cited study that the presence of hypocalcemia at parturition (defined as serum total calcium concentration $>$7.9 mg/dL) resulted in a 4.8 times greater risk of developing left displaced abomasum than dairy cattle with normal calcium concentrations[70] is confounded in that the study failed to adjust the risk for age. It has been well documented that older cattle are at markedly increased risk for developing left displaced abomasum[1] and hypocalcemia; the observed increased risk of hypocalcemic cattle for abomasal displacement in the 1993 study[70] most likely reflected the confounding effect of age.

Hypocalcemia can be treated with intravenous, subcutaneous, or oral administration of calcium solutions.[71] Subcutaneous administration of calcium solutions has been practiced for many years as part of the treatment of hypocalcemic cattle. To facilitate absorption, it is preferable to administer no more than 125 mL at a site, although this supposition and volume do not appear to have been verified. A 14-gauge needle is placed subcutaneously over the lateral thorax, 125 mL is administered, the needle is redirected, and another 125 mL administered. The process is then repeated on the other side of the cow. The effectiveness of subcutaneous administration of calcium gluconate in increasing serum calcium concentration has been documented in healthy cows[72] as well as pariparturient cows with clinical signs of hypocalcemia. Commercially available formulations of calcium gels typically contain 50 g of $CaCl_2$ and increase plasma calcium concentrations within 30 to 60 minutes and for at least 6 hours.[73–76] Retreatment at 12-hour intervals if needed may be indicated; 2 treatments provide 100 g of $CaCl_2$ and 37 g of calcium over 24 hours. These treatment recommendations for hypocalcemia-induced abomasal hypomotility need to be verified in a prospective randomized clinical trial.

Potassium if Hypokalemia Is Present

Cows with severe hypokalemia have profound muscle weakness leading to recumbency, decreased gastrointestinal tone, and depression.[77–79] Of interest are the results of a 1997 study that hypokalemia preceeded LDA in 3 cows,[80] and the results of a 2010 in vitro study that indicated hypokalemia decreases abomasal smooth muscle tone[16] and may therefore play a role in the development and maintenance of abomasal hypomotility and abomasal displacement. The relationship between plasma potassium concentration and smooth muscle tone has not been determined for cattle, but studies in humans suggest hypokalemia must be marked (>2.0–2.5 mEq/L) to decrease skeletal muscle tone[81]; presumably plasma potassium concentrations of this magnitude will also decrease smooth muscle tone. Because potassium depletion decreases the motility and propulsive ability of the intestine in the rat,[82] it is likely that severe hypokalemia decreases gastrointestinal motility and potentially increases the risk of developing left displaced abomasum in lactating dairy cattle. The effect of potassium appears to be due to a lack of stimuli rather than an inability of gastro-intestinal smooth muscle to respond.[82,83]

Oral potassium administration is the method of choice for treating hypokalemia. Inappetant adult cattle should be treated with at least 30 to 60 g of feed grade KCl twice at a 12-hour interval, with the KCl placed in gelatin boluses or administered by ororuminal intubation.[71] Adult cattle with severe hypokalemia (>2.5 mEq/L) should initially be treated with 120 g of KCl PO, followed by two 60-g KCl oral treatment at 8-hour intervals, for a total 24-hour treatment of approximately 240 g of KCl. Daily oral doses larger than 240 g of KCl are not recommended as they can lead to diarrhea, excessive salivation, muscular tremors of the legs, and excitability.[71] These treatment recommendations for hypokalemia-induced abomasal hypomotility need to be verified in a prospective randomized clinical trial.

INEFFECTIVE TREATMENTS FOR ABOMASAL HYPOMOTILITY

Flunixin Meglumine

In general, stimulation of sympathetic nerves decreases gastrointestinal smooth muscle tone in vivo and in vitro; such a decrease is usually accompanied by a decrease in gastrointestinal motility.[64] It is for this reason that amelioration of sympathetic nervous system activation in diseased cattle has the potential to improve gastrointestinal motility in animals with hypomotility or atony. Consequently, parenteral administration of nonsteroidal anti-inflammatory drugs has a strong theoretical background as part of the initial treatment of diseased cattle with gastrointestinal hypomotility. Unfortunately, the results of 3 clinical studies indicate that flunixin meglumine does not have any prokinetic activity in promoting abomasal emptying rate when administered preoperatively to cows with left displaced abomasum.[5,31,33] These results are consistent with those in healthy humans, where cyclooxygenase-2 inhibitors did not alter gastric emptying.[84] The result of one study in cattle with left displaced abomasum[5] administered flunixin meglumine or erythromycin was discussed previously. Two other clinical trials have been conducted in cattle with left displaced abomasum that indicate flunixin meglumine does not have a prokinetic effect in cattle with abomasal hypomotility. However, because endotoxemia decreases abomasal emptying rate[11,12] and flunixin meglumine is effective in ameliorating some of the effects of endotoxin, it is possible that flunixin meglumine could be an effective prokinetic agent in cattle with endotoxin-induced abomasal hypomotility.

Forty-five dairy cows with left displaced abomasum were sequentially assigned to treatment with flunixin meglumine (2.2 mg/kg, IV; n = 15), Neoancemin (7 mL/100 kg IV, n = 15; this solution contains chlorpheniramin [12.5 mg/mL], ascorbic acid [100 mg/mL], thiamine-HCl [10 mg/mL], and glucose [100 mg/mL]), or an untreated control group (n = 15) with treatment being administered 2 hours before surgical correction was performed.[31] Administration of flunixin meglumine did not alter abomasal emptying rate in the immediate postoperative period as assessed by D-xylose absorption; however, administration of Neoancemin did increase abomasal emptying rate.[31]

In a follow-up study, 30 dairy cows with left displaced abomasum were sequentially assigned to treatment with flunixin meglumine (2.2 mg/kg, IV; n = 15) or an untreated control group (n = 15) with treatment being administered 2 hours before surgical correction was performed.[33] Administration of flunixin meglumine did not alter abomasal emptying rate in the immediate postoperative period, as assessed by D-xylose absorption but did improve the general clinical condition of the cow, as assessed by rumen contraction rate and feed intake.[33]

Dopaminergic Antagonists

Metoclopramide is an antagonist at dopaminergic (D_2) receptors and a serotonin (5-hydroxytryptamine; 5-HT) agonist at 5-HT_4 receptors and serotonin antagonist at 5-HT_3 receptors.[85] As such, metoclopramide inhibits gastric accommodation in humans and dogs, resulting in higher luminal pressures and increased rate of gastric emptying.[86] A 2003 in vitro study documented that smooth muscle from the pyloric antrum of cattle contracted upon addition of 5-HT_2 and 5-HT_4 agonists.[87] This finding suggested that metoclopramide may exert a prokinetic effect in ruminants. However, because abomasal emptying in ruminants is better characterized as fluid emptying rather than semisolid or solid emptying,[2,25,88,89] serotonergic mechanisms appear to play a less important role in antroduodenal motility than in monogastrics. This is probably due to the very low expression of 5-HT_4 receptors in the abomasum fundus and pyloric antrum in adult cattle relative to the ileum, cecum, and colon.[90,91] Moreover, a major obstacle to the use of metoclopramide in ruminants is the occurrence of dose-dependent adverse behavior. Excitement followed by depression and somnolence has been observed in cattle and goats after administration of metoclopramide at doses of 0.1 mg/kg or greater.[2,92–95] In humans, metoclopramide is a neuroleptic agent that induces extrapyramidal activity (including torticollis, opisthotonus, trismus, and facial spasms), which is more likely to occur in children.[96]

In an in vitro study using smooth muscle harvested from the pyloric antrum of healthy cattle, metoclopramide failed to demonstrate any effect on contractility.[56] Metoclopramide has been used to treat vagal indigestion of cattle[97] and abomasal emptying defect of sheep,[98] but treatment efficacy could not be evaluated in these studies because administration was not randomized and observers were not masked to treatment assignment. In a study in sheep, low metoclopramide doses (0.023 and 0.045 mg/kg, administration route not reported) did not alter myoelectrical activity or tension of the pyloric antrum in sheep.[99] In a study in adult goats, very high metoclopramide doses (0.5 mg/kg, IM or IV) did not alter the electromyographic activity of the abomasal body but transiently increased the electrical activity of the pyloric antrum.[95]

Administration of metoclopramide (0.1 mg/kg, SC) decreased antral spike rate in yearling cattle,[34] which is suggestive of decreased contractility. Metoclopramide (0.1 mg/kg, SC) facilitated, rather than inhibited, gastric accommodation in milk-fed calves, and consequently tended to slow the rate of abomasal emptying.[2] Taken together, the available evidence indicates that metoclopramide (0.1–0.2 mg/kg, IM or SC) either does not alter or slightly decreases the abomasal emptying rate in adult ruminants and milk-fed calves. Metoclopramide should not be administered at higher dose rates than 0.1 to 0.2 mg/kg IM or SC because of the occurrence of adverse behavioral effects.

Cyanocobalamin and Butafosfan

Thirty dairy cows with left displaced abomasum were assigned sequentially to treatment with Catosal (100 mg butafosfan and 50 μg cyanocobalamine per mL of solution; 5 mL/100 kg BW, IV; n = 15) or an untreated control group (n = 15) before surgical correction was performed.[32] Administration of Catosal did not alter abomasal emptying rate in the immediate postoperative period, as assessed by D-xylose absorption but did improve energy homeostasis, as assessed by plasma concentrations of nonesterified fatty acids, β-OH butyrate, and bilirubin.[32] Catosal was not hypothesized to alter abomasal motility in this study.

SUMMARY

The results of clinical trials and experimental studies are unanimous in their conclusion that the most effective prokinetic for abomasal hypomotility in cattle is erythromycin (8.8–10 mg/kg, IM). This finding is consistent with that in humans with impaired gastric hypomotility, where a systematic review indicated that erythromycin was the most effective prokinetic agent.[100] Erythromycin is an effective prokinetic in cattle with abomasal hypomotility (left displaced abomasum, abomasal volvulus) and its prokinetic effect is accompanied by clinically significant increases in milk production and rumen contraction rate.[5,6] The prokinetic effect of erythromycin is sufficiently strong to warrant a clinical trial of its use in the medical treatment of left displaced abomasum in conjunction with rolling the cow and repositioning the abomasum to the ventral midline.[5,24,89] Parenteral administration of erythromycin is labeled in the United States for treatment of pneumonia, pneumonia-enteritis complex, foot rot, metritis, and stress in beef cattle and for treatment of pneumonia, foot rot, metritis, and stress in dairy cattle. The recommended dose rate is 1.1 to 8.8 mg/kg (0.5–4 mg/lb), IM, every 24 hours, and the milk and meat withdrawal times are 3 and 14 days, respectively. Therefore, parenteral administration of erythromycin to calves and adult cattle as a prokinetic agent constitutes extra label drug use. It is clearly inappropriate to administer an antimicrobial for a nonantimicrobial effect (such as increasing abomasal emptying rate) as such use may unnecessarily promote the development of antimicrobial resistance. Two other macrolides (tylosin and tilmicosin) are also effective prokinetic drugs in healthy milk-fed calves[36] and presumably adult cattle with abomasal hypomotility, but their motility promoting effects are milder than erythromycin and have not been proven in a clinical trial of diseased cattle to be clinically significant.

The available evidence indicates that the direct acting parasympathomimetic agent bethanechol (0.07 mg/kg SC) can result in a general increase in gastrointestinal tract tone, which may not necessarily facilitate abomasal emptying. In fact, a generalized increase in intestinal smooth muscle tone may impede abomasal emptying in ruminants administered an effective prokinetic agent.[2] Parasympathomimetics cannot be currently recommended as prokinetic agents in promoting abomasal motility due to the lack of controlled clinical trials demonstrating their effectiveness. However, because some in vitro findings are supportive of a prokinetic effect, a randomized clinical trial of bethanechol versus positive control (erythromycin) and negative control (0.9% NaCl) treatments appears indicated. Such a trial should also document potential deleterious side effects of bethanechol, including increased urination, salivation, and cardiovascular effects.[54]

The available evidence suggests that calcium and potassium are likely to be effective prokinetic agents in cattle with marked hypocalcemia and hypokalemia, respectively. Randomized clinical trials appear indicated.

The available evidence indicates that metoclopramide is not an effective prokinetic drug in cattle, and its use cannot be recommended. The results of 3 clinical trials indicated that the nonsteroidal anti-inflammatory agent flunixin meglumine is not an effective treatment for abomasal hypomotility.[5,31,33]

REFERENCES

1. Constable PD, Miller GY, Hoffsis GF, et al. Risk factors for abomasal volvulus and left abomasal displacement in cattle. Am J Vet Res 1992;53:1184–92.
2. Wittek T, Constable PD. Assessment of effects of erythromycin, neostigmine, and metoclopramide on abomasal motility and emptying rate in calves. Am J Vet Res 2005;66:545–52.
3. Vlaminck K, van den Hende C, Muylle E, et al. Left-sided abomasal displacement: II Influence of some therapeutics. Vlaams Diergeneeskundig Tijdschrift 1984;53: 13–20.
4. Wittek T, Schreiber K, Furll M, et al. Use of D-xylose absorption test to measure abomasal emptying rate in healthy lactating Holstein-Friesian cows and in cows with left displaced abomasum or abomasal volvulus. J Vet Intern Med 2005;19:905–13.
5. Wittek T, Tischer K, Gieseler T, et al. Effect of preoperative administration of erythromycin or flunixin meglumine on postoperative abomasal emptying rate in dairy cows undergoing surgical correction of left displacement of the abomasum. J Am Vet Med Assoc 2008;232:418–23.
6. Wittek T, Tischer K, Körner I, et al. Effect of preoperative erythromycin or dexamethasone/vitamin C on postoperative abomasal emptying rate in dairy cows undergoing surgical correction of abomasal volvulus. Vet Surg 2008;37:537–44.

7. Daniel RCW. Motility of the rumen and abomasum during hypocalcemia. Can J Comp Med 1983;47:276–80.
8. Vlaminck K, van den Hende C, Oyaert W, et al. Left-sided abomasal displacement: Hypocalcemia as a possible cause of diminished gastro-intestinal motility. Vlaams Diergeneeskundig Tijdschrift 1984;53:4–12.
9. Madison JB, Troutt HF. Effects of hypocalcaemia on abomasal motility. Res Vet Sci 1988;44:264–6.
10. van Meirhaeghe H, Deprez P, van den Hende C, et al. The influence of insulin on abomasal emptying rate in cattle. J Vet Med A 1988;35:213–20.
11. Vlaminck K, Van Meirhaeghe HV, Den Hende C. Einfluss von Endotoxinen auf die Labmagenentleerung beim Rind. Dtsch Tierärztl Wschr 1985;92:392–5.
12. Kaze C, Mevissen M, Hirsbrunner G, et al. Effect of endotoxins on contractility of smooth muscle preparations from the bovine abomasal antrum. Dtsch tierärztl Wschr 2004;111:28–35.
13. Poulsen JSD, Jones BEV. The influence of metabolic alkalosis and other factors on abomasal emptying rate in goats and cows. Nord Vet Med 1974;26:22–30.
14. Poulsen JSD, Jones BEV. Beitrag zur Labmagenverlagerung-Einfluβ der Kalziumionen und der metabolischen Alkalose auf die-Entleerungsgeschwindigkeit des Labmagens. Dtsch Tierärztl Wschr 1974;81:562–3.
15. Holtenius K, Jacobson MSO, Holtenius P. Effects of intravenous infusion of glucose and pancreatic glucagon on abomasal function in dairy cows. Acta Vet Scand 1998;39:291–300.
16. Türck G, Leonhard-Marek S. Potassium and insulin affect the contractility of abomasal smooth muscle. J Dairy Sci 2010;93:3561–8.
17. Nouri M, Constable PD. Comparison of two oral electrolyte solutions and route of administration on the abomasal emptying rate of Holstein-Friesian calves. J Vet Intern Med 2006;20:620–62.
18. Sen I, Constable PD, Marshall TS. Effect of suckling isotonic or hypertonic solutions of sodium bicarbonate or glucose on abomasal emptying rate in calves. Am J Vet Res 2006;67:1377–84.
19. Constable PD, Grünberg W, Carstensen L. Comparative effects of two oral rehydration solutions on milk clotting, abomasal luminal pH, and abomasal emptying rate in suckling calves. J Dairy Sci 2009;92:296–312.
20. Hara S, Takahashi K, Tomizawa Y, et al. Effects of fasting and xylazine sedative on digestive tract motility, rumen VFA and certain blood components in ruminants. Veterinarija Zootechnika 2002;19(41):5–14.
21. Geishauser T, Reiche D, Schemann AM. In vitro motility disorders associated with displaced abomasum in dairy cows. Neurogastroenterol Mot 1998;10:395–401.
22. Niederberger MD, Hirsbrunner G, Steiner A, et al. In vitro effects of bethanechol on abomasal and duodenal smooth muscle preparations from dairy cows with left displacement of the abomasum from healthy dairy cows. Vet J 2010;184:88–94.
23. Steiner A, Roussel AJ. Drugs coordinating and restoring gastrointestinal motility and their effect on selected hypodynamic gastrointestinal disorders in horses and cattle. J Vet Med A 1995;42:613–31.
24. Wittek T, Constable PD, Morin DE. Ultrasonographic assessment of change in abomasal position during the last three months of gestation and first three months of lactation in Holstein-Friesian cows. J Am Vet Med Assoc 2005;227:1469–75.
25. Wittek T, Constable PD. Changes in abdominal dimensions during late gestation and early lactation in Holstein-Friesian heifers and cows and their association with left displaced abomasum. Vet Rec 2007;161:155–61.

26. Kelly KA. Gastric emptying of liquids and solids: roles of proximal and distal stomach. Am J Physiol 1980;239:G71–6.
27. Low AG. Nutritional regulation of gastric secretion, digestion, and emptying. Nutr Res Rev 1990;3:229–52.
28. Pfannkuche H, Reiche D, Hoppe S, et al. Cholinergic and noncholinergic innervation of the smooth muscle layers in the bovine abomasum. Anat Rec 2002;267:70–7.
29. Ontsouka EC, Niederberger M, Steiner A, et al. Binding sites of muscarinic and adrenergic receptors in gastrointestinal tissues of dairy cows suffering from left displacement of the abomasum. Vet J 2010;186:328–37.
30. Wittek T. A review on stimulation of abomasal motility and emptying after surgical correction of left displaced abomasum or abomasal volvulus. Prakt Tierarzt 2010; 91:892–8.
31. Gieseler T, Wittek T, Fürll M. Einfluss von Flunixin-Meglumine und Neoancemin auf die klinische Rekonvaleszens und die Labmagenentleerung bein Kühen mit linksseitiger Labmagenverlagerung. Slov Vet Res 2006;43(Suppl 10):195–7.
32. Fürll M, Wittek T, Gengenbach S, et al. Effects of preoperative application of butafosfan and cyanocobalamin on reconvalescence, clinico-chemical parameters, antioxidative metabolism and postoperative abomasal emptying in cows with abomasal dislocation. Tierärztl Prax 2006;34(G):351–6.
33. Gieseler T, Wittek T, Fürll M. Effects of preoperative flunixin meglumine in cows with left abomasal displacement (LDA). Tierärztl Prax 2008;36(G):15–9.
34. Roussel AJ, Brumbaugh GW, Waldron RC, et al. Abomasal and duodenal motility in yearling cattle after administration of prokinetic drugs. Am J Vet Res 1994;55:111–5.
35. Huhn JC, Nelson DR, Constable PD, et al. Prokinetic properties of erythromycin lactobionate in cattle. Proc XX World Buiatrics Congress 1998;177–81.
36. Nouri M, Constable PD. Effect of parenteral administration of erythromycin, tilmicosin, and tylosin on abomasal emptying rate in suckling calves. Am J Vet Res 2007;68:1392–8.
37. Nouri M, Hajikolaee MR, Constable PD, et al. Effect of erythromycin and gentamicin on abomasal emptying rate in suckling calves. J Vet Intern Med 2008;22:196–201.
38. Afshari G, Nouri M, Hassan EB, et al. Effect of parenteral administration of ivermectin and erythromycin on abomasal emptying rate in suckling calves. Am J Vet Res 2009;70:527–31.
39. Buret AG. Immuno-modulation and anti-inflammatory benefits of antibiotics: the example of tilmicosin. Can J Vet Res 2010;74:1–10.
40. Itoh Z, Nakay M, Suzuki T, et al. Erythromycin mimics exogenous motilin in gastrointestinal contractile activity in the dog. Am J Physiol 1984;247:G688–94.
41. Annese V, Jenssens J, Vantrapen G, et al. Erythromycin accelerates gastric emptying by inducing antral contractions and improved gastroduodenal coordination. Gastroenterology 1992;102:823–8.
42. Itoh Z. Motilin and clinical application. Peptides 1997;18:593–608.
43. Khiat A, Boulanger Y. Identification of the motilide pharmacophores using quantitative structure activity relationships. J Peptide Res 1998;52:321–8.
44. Xu L, Depoortere I, Vertongen P, et al. Motilin and erythromycin-A share a common binding site in the third transmembrane segment of the motilin receptor. Biochem Pharmacol 2005;70:879–87.
45. Pilot MA. Macrolides in roles beyond antibiotic therapy. Br J Surg 1994;81:1423–9.
46. Constable PD, St. Jean G, Hull BL, et al. Prognostic value of surgical and postoperative findings in cattle with abomasal volvulus. J Am Vet Med Assoc 1991;199(7): 892–8.

47. Janssens J, Peeters TL, Vantrappen G, et al. Improvement of gastric emptying in diabetic gastroparesis by erythromycin. N Engl J Med 1990;322:1028–31.
48. Depoortere I, Peeters TL, Vantrappen G. Effect of erythromycin and of octreotide on motilin receptor density in the rabbit. Regul Pept 1991;32:85–94.
49. Ontsouka EC, Bruckaimaer RM, Steiner A, et al. Messenger RNA levels and binding sites of muscarinic acetylcholine receptors in gastrointestinal muscle layers from healthy dairy cows. J Recept Signal Transd Res 2007;27:147–66.
50. Stoffel MH, Monnard CW, Steiner A, et al. Distribution of muscarinic receptor subtypes and interstitial cells of Cajal in the gastrointestinal tract of healthy dairy cows. Am J Vet Res 2006;67:1992–97.
51. Caulfield MP, Birdsall NJ. International Union of Pharmacology. XVII. Classification of muscarinic acetylcholine receptors. Pharmacol Rev 1998;50:279–90.
52. Braun U, Gansohr B, Haessig M. Ultrasonographic evaluation of reticular motility in cows after administration of atropine, scopolamine and xylazine. J Vet Med A Physiol Pathol Clin Med 2002;49:299–302.
53. Pfeiffer JB, Mevissen M, Steiner A, et al. In vitro effects of bethanechol on intestinal smooth muscle preparations from the duodenum and jejeunum of healthy dairy cows. Am J Vet Res 2007;68:313–22.
54. Buehler M, Steiner A, Meylan M, et al. In vitro effects of bethanechol on smooth muscle preparations from abomasal fundus, corpus, and antrum of dairy cows. Res Vet Sci 2008;84:441–51.
55. Zanolari P, Meylan M, Marti M, et al. In vitro effects of bethanechol on intestinal smooth muscle preparations in presence and absence of M_2 or M_3 muscarinic receptor antagonists in healthy dairy cows. Dtsch Tierärztl Wschr 2007;114:171–7.
56. Michel A, Mevissen M, Burkhardt HW, et al. In vitro effects of cisapride, metoclopramide and bethanechol on smooth muscle preparations from abomasal antrum and duodenum. J vet Pharmacol Therap 2003;26:413–20.
57. Thornton JT. Treatment of left-sided abomasal displacement. Modern Vet Pract 1970:51(5):68.
58. Olson VF, Krumm D. Treatment of right-sided abomasal displacement. Modern Vet Pract 1976;57:195.
59. Clark R, Weiss KE. Studies on the comparative actions of carbamylcholine, physostigmine and neostigmine in different species of domestic animals. Onderstepoort J Vet Res 1954;26:485–99.
60. Buchanan M, Cousin DAH, MacDonald NM, et al. Medical treatment of right-sided dilatation of the abomasum in cows. Vet Rec 1991;129:111–2.
61. Dardillat C, Ruckebusch Y. Aspects fonctionnels de la jonction gastro-duodenale chez le veau nouveau-ne. Ann Rech Veter 1973;4:31–56.
62. Smith RH. Passage of ingesta through the calf abomasum and small intestine. J Physiol 1964;172:305–20.
63. Adams SB, MacHarg MA. Neostigmine methylsulfate delays gastric emptying of particulate markers in horses. Am J Vet Res 1985;46:2498–9.
64. Meylan M, Georgieva TM, Reist M, et al. Distribution of mRNA that codes for subtypes on adrenergic receptors in gastrointestinal tract of dairy cows. Am J Vet Res 2004;65:1595–603.
65. Jang KH, Kang WM, Lee JM, et al. Electroacupuncture and moxibustion for correction of abomasal displacement in dairy cattle. Proceedings of the 27th Annual International Congress on Veterinary Acupuncture. IVAS, Canada, 2001:171–6.
66. Huber TL, Wilson RC, Stattelman AJ, et al. Effect of hypocalcemia on motility of the ruminant stomach. Am J Vet Res 1981;42:1488–90.

67. Hara S, Ikegaya Y, Jørgensen RJ, et al. Effect of induced subclinical hypocalcemia on the motility of the bovine digestive tract. Acta Vet Scand 2003;Suppl 98:251.
68. Bajcsy AC, Rehage J, Scholz H, et al. Changes in blood ionized calcium and some other blood parameters before and after replacement of a left-sided displaced abomasum in dairy cattle. Dtsch Tierärztl Wschr 1997;104:501–40.
69. LeBlanc SJ, Leslie KE, Duffield TF. Metabolic predictors of displaced abomasum in dairy cattle. J Dairy Sci 2005;88:159–70.
70. Massey CD, Wang C, Donovan GA, et al. Hypocalcemia at parturition as a risk factor for left displacement of the abomasum in dairy cows. J Am Vet Med Assoc 1993;203:852–3.
71. Constable PD. Fluids and electrolytes. Vet Clin North Am Food Anim Pract 2003: 19(3):1–40.
72. Goff JP. Treatment of calcium, phosphorus, and magnesium balance disorders. In: Roussel AJ, Constable PD. Guest Editors, Fluid and electrolyte therapy. Vet Clin North Am Food Anim Pract 1999;15(3):619–39.
73. Queen WG, Miller GY, Masterson MA. Effects of oral administration of a calcium-containing gel on serum calcium concentration in postparturient dairy cows. J Am Vet Med Assoc 1993;202:607–9.
74. Oetzel GR. Effect of calcium chloride gel treatment in dairy cows on incidence of periparturient diseases. J Am Vet Med Assoc 1996;209:958–61.
75. Dhiman TR, Sasidharan V. Effectiveness of calcium chloride in increasing blood calcium concentrations of periparturient dairy cows. J Anim Sci 1999;77:1597–605.
76. Hernandez J, Risco CA, Elliott JB. Effect of oral administration of a calcium chloride gel on blood mineral concentrations, parturient disorders, reproductive performance, and milk production of dairy cows with retained fetal membranes. J Am Vet Med Assoc 1999;215:72–6.
77. Sielman ES, Sweeney RW, Whitlock RH, et al. Hypokalemia syndrome in dairy cows: 10 cases (1992–1996). J Am Vet Med Assoc 1997;210:240–3.
78. Sattler N, Fecteau G, Girard C, et al. Description of 14 cases of bovine hypokalemia syndrome. Vet Rec 1998;143:503–7.
79. Peek SF, Divers TJ, Guard C, et al. Hypokalemia, muscle weakness, and recumbency in dairy cattle. Vet Therap 2000;1:235–44.
80. Fürll M, Bialek N, Jäkel L, et al. Displacement of the abomasum in adult cattle in east Germany: incidence, etiology, and prevention. Prakt Tierarzt Collegium Veterinarium 1997;XXVII;81–6.
81. Brobst D. Review of the pathophysiology of alterations in potassium homeostasis. J Am Vet Med Assoc 1986;188:1019–25.
82. Perdue HS, Phillips PH. Stimulation of peristalsis in the potassium deficient rat by acetyl-B-methylcholine. Proc Soc Exp Biol Med 1952;80:248–50.
83. Welt LG, Hollander W, Blythe WB. The consequences of potassium depletion. J Chron Dis 1960;11:213–54.
84. Bouras EP, Burton DD, Camilleri M, et al. Effect of cyclooxygenase-2 inhibitors on gastric emptying and small intestinal transit in humans. Neurogastroenterol Motil 2004;16:729–35.
85. Plaza MA, Arruebo MP, Murillo MD. Effects of 5-hydroxytryptamine agonists on myoelectric activity of the forestomach and antroduodenal area in sheep. J Pharm Pharmacol 1996;48:1302–8.
86. Meyer JH. Motility of the stomach and gastroduodenal junction. In Johnson LR, editor. Physiology of the gastrointestinal tract. 2nd ed. New York: Raven Press; 1987. p. 613–29.

87. Spring C, Mevissen M, Reist M, et al. Modification of spontaneous contractility of smooth muscle preparations from the bovine abomasal antrum by serotonin receptor agonists. J Vet Pharmacol Ther 2003;26:377–85.
88. Wittek T, Constable PD, Morin DE. Abomasal impaction in Holstein-Friesian cows: 80 cases (1980–2003). J Am Vet Med Assoc 2005;227:287–91.
89. Wittek T, Locher L, Alkaassem A, et al. Effect of surgical correction of left displaced abomasum by means of omentopexy via right flank laparotomy or two-step laparoscopy-guided abomasopexy on postoperative abomasal emptying rate in lactating dairy cows. J Am Vet Med Assoc 2009;234:652-7.
90. Meylan M, Georgieva TM, Reist M, et al. Distribution of mRNA that codes for 5-hydroxytryptamine receptor subtypes in the gastrointestinal tract of dairy cows. Am J Vet Res 2004;65:1151–8.
91. Ontsouka EC, Blum JW, Steiner A, et al. 5-hydroxytryptamine-4 receptor messenger ribonucleic acid levels and densities in gastrointestinal muscle layers from healthy dairy cows. J Anim Sci 2006;84:3277–84.
92. Zdelar F, Hahn V, Martinic B, et al. Effect of the antiemetic metoclopramide on the digestive tract of fattening calves, and its use in digestive disorders. Veterinarski Glasnik 1979;33:761–6.
93. Guard C, Schwark W, Kelton D, et al. Effects of metoclopramide, clenbuterol, and butorphanol on ruminoreticular motility in calves. Cornell Vet 1988;78:89–98.
94. Jones RD, Mizinga KM, Thompson FN, et al. Bioavailability and pharmacokinetics of metoclopramide in cattle. J Vet Pharmacol Ther 1994;17:141–7.
95. Huhn JC, Nelson DR. The quantitative effect of metoclopramide on abomasal and duodenal myoelectric activity of goats. J Vet Med A 1997;44:361–71.
96. Pinder RM, Brogden RN, Sawyer PR, et al. Metoclopramide: a review of its pharmacological properties and clinical use. Drugs 1976;12:81–131.
97. Braun U, Steiner A, Kaegi B. Clinical, haematological and biochemical findings and the results of treatment in cattle with acute functional pyloric stenosis. Vet Rec 1990;126:107–10.
98. Ruegg PL, George LW, East NE. Abomasal dilatation and emptying defect in a flock of Suffolk ewes. J Am Vet Med Assoc 1988;193:1534–6.
99. Kopcha M. Myoelectrical and myomechanical response of the pyloric antrum in sheep to metoclopramide. Proceedings of 6th Annual Veterinary Medical Forum of the ACVIM 1988;733.
100. Sturm A, Holtmann G, Goebell H, et al. Prokinetics in patients with gastroparesis: a systematic analysis. Digestion 1999;60:422–7.

Evidence-Based Medicine Concerning Efficacy of Vaccination Against *Clostridium chauvoei* Infection in Cattle

Francisco A. Uzal, DVM, MSc, PhD

KEYWORDS

- Evidence-based medicine • Vaccination
- *Clostridium chauvoei* • Cattle

Clostridium chauvoei causes blackleg and malignant edema in cattle, sheep, and occasionally other animal species. The organism has been blamed for other less well defined conditions (eg, "sudden death syndrome") in cattle,[1] although little, if any, evidence is available to support this claim. In cattle, blackleg is usually a disease of young animals, with most cases being observed in individuals between 2 months and 2 years of age.[2,3] *C chauvoei* is a sporulated anaerobic rod that is ubiquitous in most areas of cattle production of the world. Blackleg is considered an endogenous infection because the spores of the organism remain latent in tissues of the animals after being ingested, until a tissue injury produces anaerobiosis, allowing for germination of the spores with the consequent multiplication of the germ and production of toxins.[2,3]

Vaccination against the common clostridial diseases of cattle (including *C chauvoei* infections) has been practiced for more than 70 years.[4,5] Vaccination against *C chauvoei* forms part of the health management of most cattle-producing operations worldwide, and it is widely assumed by veterinarians and farmers alike that this procedure prevents disease and death produced by this microorganism. Results of several surveys indicate that between 87.5% and 92.5% of calves in the United States are given some form of clostridial vaccination before weaning.[6,7] The so-called 7-way clostridial vaccines (which contain *C chauvoei, Clostridium septicum, Clostridium novyi, Clostridium perfringens,* and *Clostridium sordellii* antigens) are the most common commercially available clostridial immunogens.[5] However, for several decades, immunogens against

The author has nothing to disclose.

California Animal Health and Food Safety, San Bernardino Branch, University of California, Davis, 105 West Central Avenue, San Bernardino, CA 92408, USA
E-mail address: fuzal@cahfs.ucdavis.edu

Vet Clin Food Anim 28 (2012) 71–77
doi:10.1016/j.cvfa.2011.12.006 vetfood.theclinics.com
0749-0720/12/$ – see front matter

C chauvoei and *C septicum* have been considered the minimum vaccination requirement for beef and dairy calves.[5]

Although the literature on blackleg is voluminous, and there is a relatively large number of articles describing the immune and other responses (eg, local reactions and feed consumption) of cattle to *C chauvoei* vaccination,[8] scientific evidence on the efficacy of vaccination against *C chauvoei* to prevent diseases and lethality in cattle is scant.

Tools such as evidence-based medicine (EBM) have been developed for human medicine and they have been used in veterinary medicine over the past few years.[9] This approach supports medical decisions by basing them on research data.[9] This tool should be put at the disposal of veterinarians to improve the quality of decision making. The systematic reviews or meta-analysis are the highest level of evidence from an EBM approach since they critically appraised the scientific evidence concerning a disease or a health issue.

The objective of this study is to assess the level of evidence concerning the efficacy of vaccination with *C chauvoei* immunogens to prevent infections by this microorganism in cattle.

MATERIAL AND METHODS

To establish the efficacy of vaccination against *C chauvoei* infections in cattle, a bibliographical search was performed using the online databases PubMed and CAB abstracts. The keywords "blackleg," "cattle," "*Clostridium chauvoei*," "vaccine," and "vaccination" were used for the search. Searches included all the articles produced by these databases using the keywords referred to, without a time limit. In addition, a large file of hard copies of articles on clostridial vaccination published between 1956 and 1980 (which were not listed in PubMed or CAB databases) and that had been collected during the past 30 years by the author were manually reviewed for information on *C chauvoei* vaccination efficacy.

Only controlled experimental studies were evaluated. To be eligible, the articles had to cover the effects of vaccination with a vaccine containing *C chauvoei* antigens to reduce disease and/or lethality in cattle after experimental challenge or natural exposure, and a control nonvaccinated group had to be included. Only in vivo studies on cattle were considered in order to offer a concrete answer for veterinarians who wish to evaluate the benefits of vaccination in prevention of *C chauvoei* infections in cattle. Studies evaluating any effect other than those of clinical disease or lethality (eg, antibody titers, body weight, or feed consumption) were excluded. Studies evaluating the effect of *C chauvoei* vaccination in vitro or in vivo in animal species other than cattle (eg, guinea pigs, sheep, or mice) were also excluded.

Every article was assessed using an arbitrary score based on duration of the trial, number of animals, parameters measured, evaluation methods, and results (**Table 1**).[10] For each study, a 100-point scale was used (**Table 1**). It was also decided that a study whose quality score was lower than 60% would be deemed of low quality. A score between 60% and 70% would indicate moderate quality, and a score of 70% or more was considered high quality. The different studies, their methodology, and their scores are summarized in **Table 1**.

RESULTS

A total of 34 articles were found by using the keywords "blackleg," "cattle," "*Clostridium chauvoei*," "vaccine," and "vaccination." Of these, only 5 articles described experimental studies[1,11–14]; these 5 articles were evaluated in the current study (**Table 1**). The 5 articles used for this study were written in English; no experimental studies were available in other languages. Of these 5 articles, 2 were considered of poor quality (score of 50 for each)[1,13]; 1 was of moderate quality (score of 70)[11]; and 2 were of high quality (score of 85 for each)[12,14] (**Table 1**).

The 5 experimental studies tested the efficacy of *C chauvoei* bacterins to prevent disease/death by this microorganism. However, only 4 of these studies[11–14] evaluated the efficacy of *C chauvoei* vaccination to prevent blackleg. The fifth article described a clinical trial to evaluate the efficacy of this vaccination to prevent the "sudden death syndrome."[1] Only 3 of the studies[12–14] evaluated the efficacy of vaccination against experimental challenge, while the other 2[1,11] relied on natural exposure, comparing mortality rate on vaccinated animals with that of unvaccinated controls. **Table 1** outlines the results of this study, presenting every article that was retained for this study. The 3 studies that used experimental challenge[12–14] had agreement that the efficacy of vaccination conferred close to 100% protection to vaccinated animals. However, there were no published studies comparing vaccination efficacy at different ages or comparing 1 dose to 2 or more. No comparison between monovalent and polyvalent vaccines was found either. Only 1 article[14] described the duration of protection—this article reported 100% protection to challenge 6 months after immunization, while after that the protection was progressively reduced to reach 50% at 12 months after vaccination.

DISCUSSION

During our search of the literature, we found a relatively large number of articles describing development and in vitro evaluation of vaccines against *C chauvoei*, as well as a relatively large number of articles describing the evaluation of these vaccines in vivo in cattle and other animal species by measuring antibody titers and other features such as local reactions and feed consumption were found. However, it was striking the small number of articles that actually described clinical trials evaluating in vivo vaccine efficacy to prevent disease and/or lethality in cattle. Most studies published show that vaccination with *C chauvoei* vaccines are 100% (or close to 100%) efficacious to prevent blackleg after natural exposure. However, the efficacy of vaccination to prevent blackleg after experimental challenge may be between 50% and 100% depending on the dose of the inocula. It is important to stress, however, that only 2 of the articles evaluated were rated as being of high quality[12,14] and 1 was rated as being of moderate quality.[11] The other 2 articles were rated as being of poor quality.[1,13]

Clostridial vaccines have historically been administered to nursing calves around branding time, when calves are first processed (eg, identified and castrated), usually at 1 to 4 months of age.[15] Rarely, clostridial vaccines are administered at birth. However, it has been suggested that vaccinating calves at this early age has several problems, including that (1) colostral immunity may be present until 1 to 6 months of age, thus negating clostridial immunization in some calves,[15] and (2) repeat vaccination (which is recommended 2–6 weeks after initial vaccination[15]) is usually not practiced. We could not find any experimental study testing the efficacy of *C chauvoei* vaccination at birth. Most commercial vaccine manufacturers recommend vaccination of calves starting at 2 months of age with a booster between 4 and 6 weeks later. We could not find, however, any experimental studies comparing the effect of vaccination (to prevent disease and/or lethality) at different ages and/or 1 dose versus 2 doses.

It has also been stated that a booster vaccination for *C chauvoei* near the time of weaning reportedly provides protection until age immunity takes over at approximately 2 years of age.[15] However, we could not find any published study comparing

Table 1
Evaluation of level of evidence of the clinical trials for each article

Immunogen	Control	Reference	Duration of Trial	Number of Animals	Challenge	Parameters Measured	Evaluation Methods	Results	Score
Multivalent bacterin-toxoid (*C chauvoei*, *C septicum*, *C novyi*, *C sordellii*, *C perfringens* types C and D); 2 doses, 28–113 days apart	Animals receiving only 1 dose of vaccine; historic records of feedlot	De Groot et al, 1997	90 days	Two doses: 35,000 One dose: 48,150	Natural exposure	Mortality	Kappa statistic	Sudden death syndrome mortality was not different in animals vaccinated with 1 or 2 doses or from the historic records of the feedlot	50
Multivalent bacterin-toxoid (*C chauvoei*, *C septicum*, *C novyi*, *C sordellii*, *C perfringens* types C and D; oil adjuvanted); 1 dose at arrival to feedlot	Animals vaccinated 14 days after arrival to feedlot	Richeson et al, 2011	56 days	Vaccine on arrival: 65 Vaccine delayed: 65	Natural exposure	Morbidity/mortality	PROC mixed procedure	No difference in morbidity or mortality was observed in animals	70

(*continued on next page*)

Table 1
(continued)

Immunogen	Control	Reference	Duration of Trial	Number of Animals	Challenge	Parameters Measured	Evaluation Methods	Results	Score
C chauvoei and *C septicum* bacterin; 1 dose	Nonvaccinated animals	Mechak et al, 1972	69 days	Vaccinated: 89 Nonvaccinated: 12	Intramuscular inoculation of *C chauvoei* spores 69 days after vaccination	Mortality	No statistical analysis performed	Vaccinated cattle challenged with C. chauvoei 69 days after vaccination showed 100% protection. Nonvaccinated cattle showed 17% protection	85
C chauvoei bacterin; number of doses not reported	Not reported	Reed & Reynolds, 1977	Not reported	Not reported	Inoculation with *C chauvoei*, route not reported	Mortality	No statistical analysis performed	Vaccinated cattle showed 100% protection	50
C chauvoei bacterins; 2 doses 4 weeks apart	Not reported	Cameron et al, 1986	6 mo 9 mo 12 mo	15 15 15	Intramuscular inoculation of *C chauvoei* spores 6, 9, or 12 mo after vaccination	Mortality	No statistical analysis performed	50%–100% protection in the 3 groups	85

Scores: <60 = low quality; 60–70, moderate quality; >70, high quality.

the duration of the protection (measured in terms of disease/lethality prevention) in animals that received a booster of *C chauvoei* vaccination at weaning. We are also unaware of published studies of the effect of calf age on response to clostridial vaccines.

This article also shows that the usefulness of EBM is frequently limited by the lack of rigorous, randomized, and controlled trials and the low number of individuals studied in many of them. This brings up the issue of anecdotal evidence versus EBM. The efficacy of clostridial vaccination to prevent blackleg in cattle is probably one of the most obvious examples in which anecdotal evidence seems to surpass scientific evidence; while almost every veterinarian and farmer in the world supports the claim that vaccination with *C chauvoei* vaccines protects cattle against blackleg, there seems to be little scientific evidence to support this claim. Collection of data on causes of disease/lethality of blackleg in vaccinated and unvaccinated cattle would help in determining the efficacy of vaccination to prevent this disease.

It would be advantageous to put tools such as EBM at the disposal of practitioners. Training in EBM during the veterinary course would be highly desirable as it would allow veterinarians to evaluate the rigor and method of systematic reviews.

REFERENCES

1. De Groot BD, Dewey CE, Griffin DD, et al. Effect of booster vaccination with a multivalent clostridial bacterin-toxoid on sudden death syndrome mortality rate among feedlot cattle. J Am Vet Med Assoc 1997;211:749–53.
2. Useh NM, Nok AJ, Esievo KA. Pathogenesis and pathology of blackleg in ruminants: the role of toxins and neuraminidase. A short review. Vet Q 2003;25:155–9.
3. Uzal FA, Paramidani M, Assis R, et al. Outbreak of clostridial myocarditis in calves. Vet Rec 2003;152:134–6.
4. Stokka GL, Edwards AJ, Spire MF, et al. Inflammatory response to clostridial vaccines in feedlot cattle. J Am Vet Med Assoc 1994;204:415–9.
5. Rogers GM, Swecker WS. Clostridial vaccines: timing and quality assurance. Comp Food Anim Med Manag 1997;19:278–85.
6. Wittum TE, Salman MD, Curtis CR, et al. The national animal health monitoring system for Colorado beef herds: management practices and their association with disease rates. Prev Vet Med 1990;8:215–25.
7. Purdy CW, Loan RW, Popham TW. Feeder calf vaccination management in seven southeastern states. AgriPract 1987;8:16–20.
8. Schipper IA, Kelling CL, Mayer J, et al. Effects of passive immunity on immune response in calves vaccinated against Clostridium chauvoei infection (blackleg). Agri Pract 1987;8:1564–6.
9. Cockcroft P, Holmes M. Handbook of evidence-based veterinary medicine. Oxford: Blackwell; 2003.
10. Vandeweerd JM, Clegg P, Buczinski S. Using systematic review to critically appraise the scientific information for the bovine veterinarian. Vet Clin North Am Food Anim Pract. In press.
11. Richeson JT, Kegley EB, Gadberry MS, et al. Effects of on arrival versus delayed clostridial or modified live respiratory vaccinations on health, performance, bovine viral diarrhea virus type I titers, and stress and immune measures of newly received beef calves. J Anim Sci 2009;87:2409–18.

12. Macheak ME, Claus KD, Maloy SE. Potency testing *Clostridium chauvoei* containing bacterins: relationship of agglutination titers and potency tests in cattle. Am J Vet Res 1972;33:1053–8.
13. Reed GA, Reynolds L. Failure of Clostridium chauvoei vaccines to protect against blackleg. Aust Vet J 1977;53:393.
14. Cameron CM, Botha WJS, Schoeman JH. Immunization of guinea pigs and cattle with a reduced dose of *Clostridium chauvoei* vaccine produced in semi-synthetic medium. Onderstepoort J Vet Res 1986;53:51–3.
15. Hjerpe CA. Bovine vaccines and herd vaccination programs. Vet Clin North Am Food Anim Pract 1990;6:171–261.

Therapeutic Efficiency of Antibiotics and Prostaglandin $F_{2\alpha}$ in Postpartum Dairy Cows with Clinical Endometritis: An Evidence-Based Evaluation

Rejean C. Lefebvre, DMV, PhD*, Angelika E. Stock, DMV, PhD

KEYWORDS

- Dairy cows • Clinical endometritis • Antibiotics
- Prostaglandin $F_{2\alpha}$

In the past decade, the decreasing fertility of dairy cows has caught considerable attention in veterinary science.[1] Since reproductive performance is strongly related to the health status of the uterus at the end of the voluntary waiting period,[2] the assessment, the treatment, and the prevention of uterine pathologies in postpartum cows have lately been the focus of research. In cows, lochia (normal postpartum discharge) is usually expelled from the reproductive tract during the first 3 weeks after parturition.[3] In some circumstances, discharges from the genital tract can persist for a variable amount of time depending on the type of organism, the cow's innate immunity, and predisposing factors to uterine diseases.[4] Uterine disease affects about half of dairy cows in the postpartum period[5,6] and causes infertility by disrupting uterine and ovarian functions.[7] Uterine inflammation is normal during the early physiologic stage of uterine involution. However, defining rigorous criteria for the diagnosis, the treatment, and the prevention of endometritis post partum remains a challenge.

Studies have used nonvalidated diagnostic criteria for endometritis, which may have jeopardized the researchers' ability to discern a true treatment effect. A new

---

The authors have nothing to disclose.
Département des Sciences Cliniques, Faculté de Médecine Vétérinaire, Saint-Hyacinthe, Université de Montréal, 3200 rue Sicotte, CP 5000, Saint-Hyacinthe, Québec, Canada, J2S 7C5
* Corresponding author.
E-mail address: rejean.lefebvre@umontreal.ca

Vet Clin Food Anim 28 (2012) 79–96
doi:10.1016/j.cvfa.2012.01.002 vetfood.theclinics.com
0749-0720/12/$ – see front matter

definition for clinical endometritis reflecting more accurately the clinical situation was proposed by Sheldon and coworkers.[2] Clinical endometritis was defined as the inflammation of the endometrium in a normal-sized uterus associated with vaginal purulent discharge after 21 DIM (days in milk) in the absence of systemic clinical disease. Purulent vaginal discharge is generally associated with *A pyogenes* infection in the uterus beyond 21 days postpartum,[7] and clinical endometritis was clearly related to a prevalence of *A pyogenes* in a different report.[9] Even though vaginal discharge is an indirect method to diagnose inflammation and infection of the uterus, the presence of purulent discharge in the anterior vagina or cervix has been consistently associated with reduced fertility in dairy cows.[10–14] The negative impact of clinical endometritis on reproductive performance is reflected by the increase of the number of services per conception, the calving–to–first service and calving–to–conception intervals,[15,16] and the reduced risk of pregnancy[17] and conception.[18] The reproductive inefficiency associated with clinical endometritis[19] translates into a significant economic loss for the dairy industry.[16,20] The financial impact is caused by excessive culling, milk loss, infertility treatment costs, and the genetic losses due to fewer replacement heifers.

Currently, 2 major therapeutic options are used for the treatment and prevention of clinical endometritis: the use of antibiotics (intrauterine or systemic) or prostaglandins ($PGF_{2\alpha}$, systemically). Antibiotics reduce the load of bacteria in the uterus and the inflammation of the endometrium.[21] The injection of $PGF_{2\alpha}$ causes luteolysis of the corpus luteum and induces estrus with increased uterine contractility and subsequent clearance of the uterine cavity. During the estrous period, local immunity prepares a better uterine environment to support embryo development and the establishment of a pregnancy. Although many reports on the subject can be found in the literature, treatment protocols for clinical endometritis are quite variable among veterinarians. The lack of negative controls, a small number of animals per treatment, different case definitions, and the use of outcome parameters based on clinical cure instead of reproductive performance make it difficult to assess the best therapeutic approach based on the available literature. By identifying, evaluating, and summarizing the best available data based on superior scientific methods, the evidence-based analysis reflects the best strategy by which to make a valid clinical decision.

OBJECTIVE

The objective of this systematic review was to analyze and summarize the results of studies with the best available evidence concerning the efficiency of different antibiotics and $PGF_{2\alpha}$ for the treatment of clinical endometritis in postpartum dairy cows. Evidence was based on subsequent reproductive performance parameters (see Types of Outcomes).

MATERIAL AND METHODS

Types of Studies

Studies using meta-analysis and controlled clinical trials were analyzed in which postpartum dairy cows were randomly allocated to different treatments of antibiotics and/or $PGF_{2\alpha}$.

Types of Interventions

Only trials comparing different antibiotics and/or $PGF_{2\alpha}$ regimens including but not limited to different drugs/different route of administration (systemically and intrauterine infusion)/duration of therapy/time of administration after calving), hormonal profile, and negative control group (untreated animals with clinical endometritis) were used. Animals included in the studies were diagnosed with clinical endometritis based on the characteristic of the postpartum vaginal discharge and the absence of systemic clinical signs of illness. In all cows, vaginal discharge was confirmed on genital examination using Metricheck (SimcroTech, Hamilton, New Zealand) or vaginoscopy.

Types of Outcomes

Trials using the following outcomes were considered: (1) improved reproductive efficiency (cumulative conception and pregnancy risk, first service conception or pregnancy risk, number of inseminations per pregnancy, hazard risk for pregnancy, calving–to–first insemination interval, calving–to–first conception interval, or calving interval and resolution risk); (2) therapeutic failure (no effect); and (3) complications (negative response to the treatment).

Search Strategy

The web search was performed using CAB and MEDLINE databases (1975–2011) with the following search terms: uterine disease, uterine infection, endometritis, clinical endometritis, bovine, cow, dairy cow, milking cow, treatment, therapy, antibiotics, prostaglandins, systemic and local treatments, intrauterine infusion, anti inflammatory drugs. Using the PubMed database, the search was based on the following keywords: endometritis, uterine infection, treatment, and cows. In addition, the reference lists of several articles on clinical endometritis were reviewed for possible additional studies.

Relevant Studies

From the databases, abstracts were assessed based on their relevant titles. Titles including words like antibiotics, specific names of antibiotics, prostaglandins, specific names of prostaglandins, uterus, postpartum, treatment effect, and cows were retained for further reading of the abstract. In the case where no abstract was available, the full article was obtained and briefly read. Studies had to reflect a meta-analysis or consist of a randomized controlled trial assessing the efficiency of antibiotics (administered systemically or by intrauterine infusion) and/or $PGF_{2\alpha}$ (administered systemically) on clinical endometritis in postpartum dairy cows. In addition, the selected studies had to present similar case definitions to qualify for the review: cows had to be presented for treatment before 45 days postpartum without systemic signs of disease. The vaginal discharge had to be diagnosed by vaginoscopy or by the use of Metricheck.

Data Collection and Analysis

From the different articles retained for critical appraisal, information about country, type of population, group size, drug regimen (drug, dose, route of administration, duration and time of treatment), diagnostic methods, follow-up and losses of animals, year of the study, exclusion or inclusion criteria for clinical endometritis, randomization and masking methods, and statistical analysis was extracted and resumed. Potential conflict of interest was recorded. Studies were evaluated for methodologic quality using the CHALMER scoring system (100 points) based on criteria of adequacy of allocation concealment on randomized clinical trials.[22]

RESULTS

Relevant Studies

Fig. 1 shows a chart of the study selection process. A total of 294 articles were found using the search strategy of the present paper. After the exclusion of most articles by title, 43 papers remained for review. Ten articles were excluded for absence of negative control, 8 for outcome measurements other than reproductive performance parameters, 6 for using a different case definition of clinical endometritis, 4 for not using a randomized treatment allocation, 2 for testing therapeutic efficiency of substances other than an antibiotic or $PGF_{2\alpha}$, 1 for a different study population of cows (buffalo cows), 1 because most of the vaginal discharge observation was based on the farmer's observations rather than on the vaginal examination (the capacity of detecting purulent discharge is higher using vaginoscopy than a simple observation[23]), 1 for incapacity to differentiate the main effect of treatment, and, finally, 1 for the use of chloramphenicol, an antibiotic that is no longer permitted to be used in food animal. Thus, only 9 studies met the inclusion criteria. From these studies, 2 articles examined the effect of $PGF_{2\alpha}$, 3 looked specifically at the effect of antibiotics, and 4 examined the effect of both antibiotics and $PGF_{2\alpha}$.

General Risk of Bias

Although studied populations from the selected articles were dairy cows, the breed was only reported in 6 (66%) studies from which the Holstein breed was most prevalent. Studies were performed in 6 different countries and using 2 different milk production systems. The annual calving system with high producing cows in North America and Europe contrasts with the seasonal calving system with pasture-based nutrition and lower producing cows in Australia and New Zealand. Both systems may differ in terms of risk factors for uterine diseases.

Cows were randomly allocated to treatment group in all studies. However, only 6 studies (66%[1,24–28]) reported a well-described method of randomization. The randomization methods used were computer-generated random number lists, tossed coins, and tag numbers (odds and pair numbers or alternate ranking numbers). An important risk of bias for all studies was the absence of a masking effect. The lack of a masking effect has a major impact on the CHALMER assessment score. The mean CHALMER score for the 9 articles was below 60% and 4 articles (44%) were below 40%. Only 1 study[13] mentioned that the team responsible for establishing the diagnosis was not aware of the treatment. All selected studies included a negative control group in the experimental design. However, the lack of follow-up examinations of animals was noticed in most studies. Only 3 clinical trials discussed some of this aspect.[24,25,27] Two studies[13,24] were funded by the pharmaceutical company of the drug used to treat endometritis. The potential conflict of interest was not discussed in these studies. Five (55%) of 9 publications did not mention any source of financial support (money, materials, drugs, etc).

Tables 1 and **2** summarize the selected papers. Studies were controlled and randomized clinical trials with negative controls (animals with clinical endometritis remained untreated).

Treatment Efficiency

Readers are referred to **Tables 3** and **4** for a summary of the results. In the 9 selected studies, 6 different antibiotics (cephapirin benzathine [CB] 500 mg intrauterine (IU); Metricure, Intervet, Australia), ceftiofur (crystalline free acid 6.6 mg/kg subcutaneous; Excede, Pfizer Animal Health, Kirkland, Québec, Canada; and hydrochloride125 mg

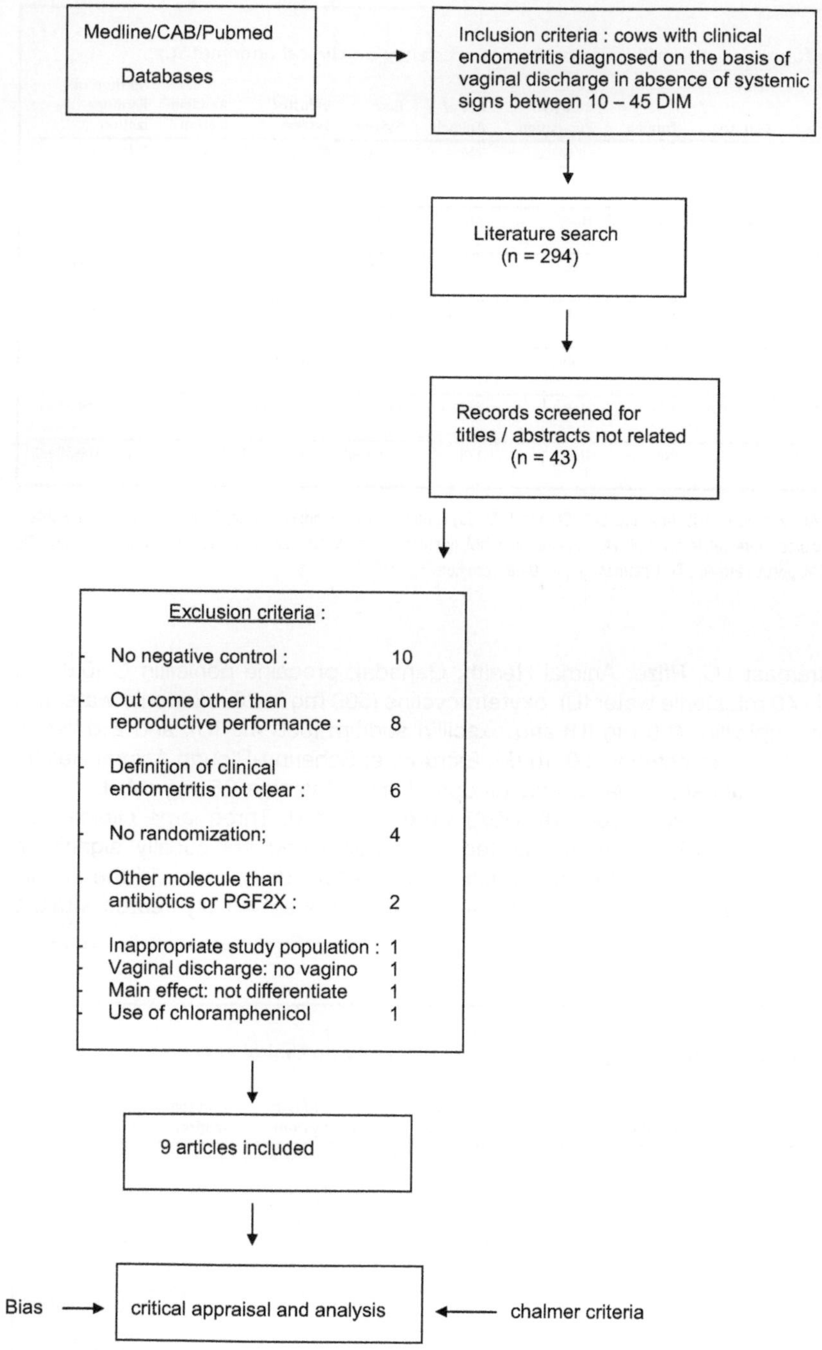

Fig. 1. Flow diagram for systemic review on the effect of antibiotics and PGF2x on reproductive performance in postpartum dairy cows with clinical endometritis.

Table 1
General information on antibiotics treatment efficiency on clinical endometritis

Authors	Year	Country	Funded	Study Population	No. of Animals	Barn System	Industry System	Random-ization	Method of Random-ization
Thurmond et al[28]	1993	USA	NM	NM	300	Freestall	Nonseasonal	Yes	Y (tag No.)
Leblanc et al[24]	2002	CAN	Intervet SP	Hols	316	Freestall	Nonseasonal	Yes	Y (computer)
Runciman et al[27]	2008	AUS	PP	NM	1325	Pasture	Seasonal	Yes	Y (second cow)
Runciman et al[14]	2009	AUS	NM	NM	326 and 113/tx	Pasture	Seasonal	Yes	y (coin toss)
Galvao et al[9]	2008	USA	NM	Hols	547	Freestall	Nonseasonal	Yes	Y (nonspecified)
Dubuc et al[13]	2010	CAN-USA	Pfizer	Hols	2178	Freestall	Nonseasonal	Yes	Y (nonspecified)
Feldmann et al[29]	2005	Germ	NM	Hols	178	Freestall	Nonseasonal	Yes	Y (nonspecified)

Abbreviations: Atb, antibiotic; AUS, Australia; CAN, Canada; DIM, day in milk; Eng, England; Fr, France; Germ, Germany; Hols, Holstein breed or crossed breed; Intervet, Intervet SP; NA, nonapplicable; NM, not mentioned; NZ, New Zealand; Pfizer, Pfizer Animal Health; PP, postpartum; PTM, post treatment; Tx, treatment group. *Data from* Refs.[9,13,14,24–29]

IU; Spectramast LC, Pfizer Animal Health, Canada), procaine penicillin G (0.8–1.0 million U in 40 mL sterile water IU), oxytetracycline (500 mg in 20 mL sterile water IU), mixture of ampicillin (400 mg IU) and oxacillin sodium (800 mg IU), and 2 different types of $PGF_{2\alpha}$ (cloprostenol 500 μg IM, Estrumate; Schering-Plough Animal Health, Pointe Claire, Québec, Canada; and dinoprost tromethamine 25 mg IM, Lutalyse; Pharmacia Upjohn, Kalamazoo, MI, USA) were evaluated. Three large clinical trial studies evaluated CB and demonstrated a favorable and statistically significant therapeutic effect on clinical endometritis in postpartum dairy cows. In the annual calving system, cows (n = 111) with clinical endometritis were initially treated with the

Table 2
General information on prostaglandin treatment efficiency on clinical endometritis

Authors	Year Public	Country	Funded	Population	No. of Animals	Barn System	Industry System	Random-ization	Method of Random-ization
Leblanc et al[24]	2002	CAN	Intervet SP	Hols	316	Freestall	Nonseasonal	Yes	Y (computer)
Dubuc et al[13]	2010	CAN-USA	Pfizer	Hols	2178	Freestall	Nonseasonal	Yes	Y (nonspecified)
Hendricks et al[25]	2006	USA	NFH and USDA	NM	214	Freestall	Nonseasonal	Yes	Y (alternate)
Feldmann et al[29]	2005	Germ	NM	Hols	178	Freestall	Nonseasonal	Yes	Y (nonspecified)
Glanvill and Dobson[26]	1991	Eng	Leverhulme Trust	NM	180	NM	Seasonal	Yes	Y (alternate)

Abbreviations: AUS, Australia; CAN, Canada; DIM, day in milk; Eng, England; Fr, France; Germ, Germany; Hols, Holstein breed or crossed breed; Intervet, Intervet SP; NA, nonapplicable; NM, not mentioned; NZ, New Zealand; Pfizer, Pfizer Animal Health; Tx, treatment group.

Table 1
(continued)

Blind	Control Group	Time of Treatment	Atb	syst/ Infusion	PGF	#anim/ Tx	Prev/ Therapeutic	Chalmer Evalutaion RCL	Chalmer Evaluation AES
NM	Y	21 and 15 DIM	Penicillin/ oxytetracycline	infusion	N	N	therapeutic	41	40
NM	Y	20–33 DIM	Cephapirin	infusion	Y	Y	therapeutic	54	50
NM	Y	28–37 PTM	Cephapirin	infusion	N	Y	therapeutic	42	40
NM	Y	7–21 PP	Cephapirin	infusion	N	Y	therapeutic		
NM	Y	44 DIM	Ceftiofur	infusion	N	N	therapeutic	33	25
Y (partial)	Y	24, 35, and 49 DIM	Ceftiofur	SC	Y	Y	prev	52	50
NM	Y	21 DIM	Ampicillin and oxacillin	IM	Y	NO	therapeutic	30	25

intrauterine infusion of 500 mg CB enveloped by a 19.6 g ointment base (Metricure, Intervet) between 27 and 33 DIM. The treated group showed a significant shorter time to pregnancy and a 63% increase of the cumulative pregnancy risk ($P = .01$) compared to untreated cows (n = 89).[24] No improvement of reproductive performance resulted when the antibiotic was initially infused between 21 and 26 DIM. In a seasonal calving system,[27] a single CB treatment improved the proportion of cows with clinical endometritis that conceived to artificial insemination ($P = .004$) when treated between 28 and 37 days before the mating start day and with a calving-to-treatment interval of less than 4 weeks. The proportion of pregnant cows within 6 and 21 weeks of mating start date was also higher ($P = .01$ and $P = .026$, respectively),

Table 2
(continued)

Blind	Control Group	Time of Treatment	$PGF_{2\alpha}$	Syst/ Infusion	PGF	#anim/ Tx	Prev/ Therapeutic	Chalmer Evalutaion RCL	Chalmer Evalutaion AES
NM	Y	20–33 DIM	Cloprostenol	IM	Y	Y	Therapeutic	54	45
Y (partial)	Y	24, 35, and 49 DIM	Dinoprost tromethamine	IM	Y	Y	prev	52	50
NM	Y	7, 14, 22, and 35 DIM	Dinoprost tromethamine	IM	Y	Y	prev/ therapeutic	50	45
NM	Y	21 DIM	Dinoprost tromethamine	IM	Y	NO	Therapeutic	30	30
NM	Y	14–28 DIM	Dinoprost tromethamine	IM	Y	NO	Therapeutic	30	25

Table 3
Summary of the results for antibiotics

Authors	Antibiotic	Time of Treatment and Diagnosis	Results	No. of Clinical Endometritis Cases
Dubuc et al, 2010[13]	Ceftiofur crystalline free acid, 6.6 mg/kg subcutaneous	Within 24 h after calving	No effect on time to 1st service for HURD No effect on time to pregnancy regardless of P4 status for HURD	323
Galvao et al, 2009[9]	Ceftiofur 125 mg intrauterine	44 DIM	No effect on 1st service conception No effect on AHR	183
Leblanc et al, 2002[24]	Cephapirin 500 mg intrauterine	20–33 DIM	Improvement of a PR by 63% (P = .01) compared with untreated for cows in presence of CL	316
Feldman et al, 2005[29]	Ampicillin 400 mg and oxacillin 800 mg intrauterine	>21 DIM	No effect	49
Runciman et al, 2008[27]	Cephapirin 500 mg intrauterine, single treatment	>7 and <29 DIM	In MAR cows, 1AICP, 3WICP, 6WICP were improved (P = .004, .006, .016 respectively).	222
Runciman et al, 2009[14]	Cephapirin 500 mg intrauterine, single treatment	>7and <29 DIM	— Treated cows showed significantly better 1st service conception risk (P = .036) and 6WICP and 21WICP P = .015 and .026 respectively.	226
Thurmond et al, 1993[28]	Exp No. 1: penicillin (~1 million) or Exp No. 2: oxytetracycline 500 mg intrauterine	21 DIM and 10–15 DIM	— No effect of treatment	— Exp No. 1: 164 — Exp No. 2: 138

Abbreviations: AHR, adjusted hazard ratio in the first 300 DIM; CL, corpus luteum; DIM, day in milk; HURD, high uterine risk disease; MAR, modified at risk; PR, pregnancy rate; P4, progesterone; 1AICP, proportion of cows that conceived to their first service to AI; 3WICP, proportion of cows pregnant within 3 weeks of mating start date; 6WICP, proportion of cows pregnant within 6 weeks of mating start date.

Table 4
Summary of the results for PGF2α

Authors	PGF2	Time of Treat and Diagnosis	Results	No. of Clinical Endometritis
Dubuc et al, 2010[13]	Dinoprost, 25 mg, IM	35 and 49 DIM	— No effect	323
Leblanc et al, 2002[24]	Cloprostenol, 500 μg, IM	20–33 DIM	— No effect	316
Feldman et al, 2005[29]	Dinoprost, 25 mg, IM	>42 DIM	— Significant higher 1st conception risk ($P<0.05$)	51
Hendrick et al, 2006[25]	Dinoprost, 25 mg, IM	7, 14, 22, 25 with or without presynch-ovsynch	— No effect	Exp No. 1: 228 Exp No. 2: 418
Glanvill and Dobson, 1991[26]	Dinoprost, 25 mg, IM	>14 and <28 DIM	—No effect	180

Abbreviations: AHR, adjusted hazard ratio in the first 300 DIM; CL, corpus luteum; DIM, day in milk; PR, pregnancy rate.

and the first service to artificial insemination was significantly better (P = .033) in treated cows (n = 103) compared to untreated ones (n = 126).[14] In both seasonal systems studies, the resolution rate of endometritis was not analyzed; however, Leblanc and colleagues[24] reported a cure rate of 77% defined as the absence of pus 14 days after the first vaginal examination. The cure rate was not affected by the treatment of CB.

There was no advantage in using the ceftiofur molecule for treatment and prevention of clinical endometritis in postpartum dairy cows. One treatment of intrauterine infusion of 125 mg ceftiofur hydrochloride (10 mL suspension, Spectramast LC; Pfizer Animal Health) at 44 DIM did not improve the reproductive performance of cows with clinical endometritis (n = 271) diagnosed with the use of Metricheck.[9] Furthermore, the preventive treatment of ceftiofur crystalline free acid (6.6 mg/kg subcutaneous at the base of the ear, Excede within 24 hours after parturition did not significantly improve the reproductive performance of cows with clinical endometritis.[13] No positive effect was measured with the intrauterine infusion of procaine penicillin G (0.8–1.0 million units in 40 mL sterile water) and oxytetracycline (500 mg in 20 mL sterile water) at 21 and 10 to 15 DIM, respectively.[28] Intrauterine infusion of a mixture of 400 mg of ampicillin and 800 mg of oxacillin at more than 21 DIM did not show any advantage on reproductive performance in cows with clinical endometritis.[29]

From the selected studies assessing the effect of $PGF_{2\alpha}$ treatment (n = 5) on reproductive performance in postpartum cows with clinical endometritis, 4 (80%) studies showed no advantage to treat cows with prostaglandins. Only Feldman and colleagues[29] reported a significant increase in the first service conception risk when cows with clinical endometritis were treated with 2 injections of $PGF_{2\alpha}$ at a 14-day interval (>42 DIM) despite the small number of animals per treatment group in the study. One study[24] reported a negative effect on reproductive performance in postpartum cows when $PGF_{2\alpha}$ was used before 26 DIM.

DISCUSSION

The ultimate goal of treating clinical endometritis in postpartum dairy cows is to significantly improve their reproductive performance while minimizing milk and meat residue issues and, consequently, reduce economic losses. Many reports on therapeutic approaches of postpartum uterine diseases and more specifically of clinical endometritis in dairy cows are available. Yet, under scrutiny, the scientific merit of most studies seems to be compromised by the lack of precise clinical definition, inconsistencies in outcomes (bacteriologic, cytologic, and clinical cure or reproductive performance based), lack of negative controls, insufficient numbers of animals per treatment group, use of inadequate or nonvalidated diagnostic methods, disparity in the studied population, lack of randomization, and faulty experimental design. For these reasons, the value and the efficiency of the treatment of clinical endometritis are still controversial. The objective of this systematic review was to use the best relevant evidence in the literature to uncover the real effect of antibiotic and $PGF_{2\alpha}$ treatment in order to make the best possible decision about the treatment of clinical endometritis in postpartum dairy cows.

To meet the objective of the present study, the best evidence is likely to come from controlled and randomized clinical trials. Nine studies were selected to answer the present question. Even though these articles represent the most relevant source of information, they have a mean CHALMER score of less than 60% (**Tables 1** and **2**). This is mainly explained by the general lack of a masking method and placebo use in all studies. The masking technique avoids bias and ensures that each group, whether treatment or control, has an equivalent placebo effect. Therefore, the measured outcome relates to the actual treatment rather than just the act of providing the treatment. The preparation of a valid placebo and the expense of additional groups (treatments with different administration route) would have made the realization of some studies more difficult and expensive and reduce the statistical power of the studies. The masking effect allows that neither the owner of the animal nor the veterinarian knows which treatment the animal has received. One study[13] ensured that veterinarians involved in the diagnosis of the clinical endometritis were not aware of the treatment allocation. Even though none of the selected studies used a systematic masking method, the CHALMER scoring system most likely underestimates the scientific value of some of the studies. For example, the large number of treated animals makes it usually difficult for farmers or veterinarian to remember the treatment administered to a specific cow. Of course, studies with a small number of animals[26,29] would have benefited from the use of a systematic masking method to reduce this bias. The no treatment control group in the experimental design ensures that the outcome does not only reflect the natural course of the disease regardless of the treatment. In the present situation, the first service conception risk would be the best outcome parameter to test the treatment effect. All selected studies in the present analysis have a control group to meet the inclusion criteria. An additional strength is the use of similar case definition and population of cows ensuring uniformity and reducing of selection bias. The choice of these criteria facilitated assessments and comparisons of results. In 4 studies, no information was available on animals that left the trial, so a systematic migration bias could not be evaluated. Finally, all studies used a random allocation, which is the most powerful method to eliminate confounding variables and to increase the probability that the measured outcome truly reflects the treatment effect. All together, these factors strengthen the present methodology for establishment of a strong cause-and-effect relationship between the treatment and the outcome (the reproductive performance). Funding could also be an important source of bias. Two studies[13,24] were funded by companies that commercialized the treatment product, and others[14,27] were partially sponsored by providing drugs or material. Despite this potential biases, negative results or absence of effects of the drug that would work against the manufacturer's interest were reported and discussed. Providing products by the industry is common in clinical research but usually represents a very small portion of the overall budget of the research project. Some studies (3 of 9) did not include this risk of bias since they did not reveal that kind of information.

Efficiency of Antibiotics

The efficiency of several antibiotics (CB, ceftiofur, penicillin G, oxacillin, oxytetracycline, and ampicillin) has been reviewed for the treatment of clinical endometritis. The rationale behind this therapeutic approach is to reduce the number of pathogens in the uterine cavity and consequently mitigate the associated inflammation, enhance the local immune defense, and facilitate the repair of the endometrium for a faster return to a normal uterine status. The CB is a first-generation cephalosporin and the only drug approved for intrauterine therapy in dairy cows. It has a 2-day meat withdrawal but no withdrawal for milk. It is effective against *A pyogenes*, the most prevalent pathogen involved in clinical endometritis.[8,9] Intrauterine administration of antibiotics is expected to reach a higher antibiotic concentration in the endometrium compared to systemic administration.[21] Clinically, CB reduces the prevalence of discharges apparent at the external cervical orifice (clinical cure) and bacteria (bacteriologic cure) in the uterus.[23]

A large portion of cows with clinical endometritis cure spontaneously without treatment. Cure rate of 77%[24] and 63%[13] as defined by the absence of vaginal purulent discharge 14 and 21 days, respectively, after the first examination was reported. A similar result (75% spontaneous resolution rate) was shown by Gautam and colleagues[30] and by Feldmann and colleagues[29] at 57.1%. The high cure rate reflects most likely the natural processes of healing during the uterine involution and may minimize the need for treatment of clinical endometritis. However, spontaneous cure of vaginal discharge does not imply increased reproductive performance and return to normal fertility. The resolution of vaginal discharge was not associated with pregnancy rate and not affected by treatment in the Canadian studies.[13,24] Thus, the need for a treatment of the condition should not be underestimated.

Three clinical trials studied the efficacy of CB as intrauterine treatment of clinical endometritis based on the improvement of the reproductive performance. Even though there was no effect of treatment with intrauterine CB on primary reproductive performance, treatment of cows with clinical endometritis initiated between 27 and 33 DIM shortened the time to the establishment of pregnancy ($P<.05$) and increased significantly the pregnancy risk relative to untreated cows.[24] Since there is uncertainty about the number of treatments received by each cow, the main effect may not have been associated with only the first treatment given between 27 and 33 DIM. This may also explain the fact that the significant effect of CB on the pregnancy rate seemed at least partly influenced by events occurring over a long period (100 days) after the first treatment (survival curve). In addition, there was a lack of association between treatment and time of enrollment ($P = .59$) in the general model. As with the Canadian study, Runciman and coworkers[26] showed no simple effect of treatment with CB on primary reproductive performance indices. However, in contrast to the annual calving system, there was a strong interaction between treatment and calving–to–treatment interval in the seasonal studies in Australia.[14,27] A single CB intrauterine infusion (500 mg) administered to cows between 28 and 37 days before the mating START date (MSD) and less than 28 days calving–to–treatment interval improved significantly the proportion of cows with clinical endometritis that conceived at the first service of artificial insemination ($P = .036$; 95% confidence interval, 1.05–3.68; odds ratio, 1.96).[14] Because of the short interval between treatment and the outcome, the first service conception risk is the reliable reproductive performance parameter to measure the efficacy of the postpartum treatment. In cows at risk of clinical endometritis following periparturient diseases with a calving–to–treatment interval less than 28 days, the treatment with CB also improved significantly the proportion of cows that conceived at first artificial insemination compared to untreated cows ($P = .004$; 95% confidence interval, 1.45–6.62; odds ratio, 3.08).[27] In both Australian studies, the sample size was calculated and only one treatment of intrauterine infusion of CB was performed. No effect of the treatment with CB was measured after 29 DIM. Although ovarian structures effect at treatment of clinical endometritis were assessed, possible hormonal effects were not analyzed.[27] Conflicting results are present concerning the calving–to–treatment interval (degree of uterine involution) and the presence of a functional corpus luteum (presence of progesterone) for the treatment of clinical endometritis. These 2 factors are physiologic variables that could account as confounders for the effect of treatment. In the seasonal calving system study,[27] 61% of the cows examined and treated ($n = 384$) before 34 DIM were between 7 and 28 DIM.[27] In this early time in the postpartum period, lochia could be difficult to distinguish from vaginal discharge associated with clinical endometritis and could confound the outcome and thus the treatment effect. Yet, a strong advantage of treating cows with clinical endometritis before 28 DIM was shown.[14,27] The presence of a corpus luteum could also be a modifier of the treatment's response as steroids can affect the cow's local immunity. Progesterone suppresses the immune response and makes the uterus more susceptible to bacterial infection.[31] Progesterone also suppresses the immune response to lipopolysaccharides in endometrial cells in vitro.[32] Most likely, the majority of high producing dairy cows are not cycling before 29 DIM and are therefore less likely to have a functional corpus luteum. Furthermore, based on progesterone levels, about 25% and 54% of high producing dairy cows have a functional corpus luteum at 12 and 49 DIM, respectively.[9] This raises a question about the real confounding value of the presence of a functional corpus luteum. In one study, the effect of intrauterine CB on cows with clinical endometritis was enhanced in the presence of a corpus luteum[24]; however, the presence of a corpus luteum was diagnosed by transrectal palpation and not confirmed by progesterone measurements. The sensitivity and specificity of rectal palpation evaluating the presence of a functional corpus luteum were 83% and 53%, respectively, compared to a rapid progesterone enzyme immunoassay with 90% and 84% sensitivity and specificity, respectively, for predicting the presence of a functional corpus luteum.[33] Bicalho and coworkers[34] reported an overall accuracy ranging from 57% to 70% to identify a functional corpus luteum by transrectal palpation. Therefore, the positive effect of CB treatment on cows with clinical endometritis between 27 and 34 DIM compared to the 21 to 26 DIM interval may not be necessarily associated with the presence of a functional corpus luteum alone. In the Australian studies, progesterone levels were not measured and the effect of P4 could therefore not be assessed. Thus, the effect of the calving–to–treatment interval and the presence of P4 on the efficacy of CB treatment of clinical endometritis remains unclear.

Single intrauterine infusions with several other antibiotics in postpartum cows with clinical endometritis were reported. Procaine penicillin G (21 DIM, 1 million units in 40 mL sterile water[28]), oxytetracycline (10–15 DIM, 500 mg in 20 mL sterile water[28]), ceftiofur hydrochloride (44 DIM, 125 mg[9]), and ampicillin (>21 DIM, 400 mg with oxacillin 800 mg[29]) were not efficient to improve reproductive performance of treated cows compared to untreated cows with clinical endometritis. Procaine penicillin G is sensitive to pencillinase enzymes secreted by bacteria that are usually present in the uterus during the early postpartum period. Bacteria like *A pyogenes* that harbor multiple virulent factors exhibit resistance to penicillin and oxytetracycline.[35] Little is known regarding the clinical efficiency of procaine penicillin G as intrauterine treatment with regard to its pharmacokinetics such as minimum inhibitory concentration and tissue diffusion. Oxytetracycline has been used by veterinarians as intrauterine antibiotic treatment in cows with clinical endometritis for a long time. However, intrauterine absorption of oxytetracycline is poor and represents a considerable risk for meat and milk residues in addition to the irritation and coagulation necrosis that are caused to the endometrium.[36,37] Thus, this antibiotic may not be very efficient and may damage the endometrium's defense mechanism and therefore even delay healing. This could explain the lack of effect of these antibiotics in the present analysis. No power-size calculation (number of animals per treatment group) was performed prior to the study. Ceftiofur hydrochloride (125 mg) is a broad-spectrum third-generation cephalosporin and is occasionally infused by veterinarian into the uterus of cows to treat clinical endometritis. Even though the intrauterine ceftiofur treatment at 44 DIM induced a bacteriologic cure, it did not influence the reproductive performance of cows with clinical endometritis compared to untreated animals.[9] Unfortunately, the use of $PGF_{2\alpha}$ (confounding factor) in a synchronization program while treating cows with ceftiofur and the lack of progesterone level assessment in this study do not allow for a critical evaluation of the effects of the uterine treatment on reproductive performance. The use of a product that is developed for mammary gland treatment as intrauterine treatment adds more uncertainty to the results because the exact minimum inhibitory concentration requirements for *A pyogenes* in uterus remain unknown. Finally, the use of ampicillin and oxacillin as intrauterine therapy for clinical endometritis in the German study did not prove to be an effective treatment of the uterine pathology.[29] Small numbers of cows per treatment groups (62–87 cows) and the absence of a power-size calculation before performing the study with these antibiotics are weak points in the trial.

Only one study assessed a preventive therapeutic approach with antibiotic by using ceftiofur crystalline free acid to prevent clinical endometritis in postpartum cows. The antibiotic was injected within 24 hours after calving in cows with higher risk for postpartum diseases.[13] Even with a total of 2178 cows, treatment with ceftiofur crystalline free acid had no effect on reproductive performance of cows with clinical endometritis compared to untreated cows. This result is surprising since a single subcutaneous administration of ceftiofur crystalline free acid (6.6 mg/kg body weight) established concentrations of the antibiotic in serum, endometrial tissue, and lochia of healthy puerperal dairy cows above the minimum inhibitory concentration of common uterine pathogens including *A pyogenes* over a 5-day period.[38] Ceftiofur crystalline free acid is known as a very effective antibiotic against most gram-positive (including *A pyogenes*) and gram-negative pathogens.[39] However, the long period between the treatment and the evaluation of the outcome in Dubuc and colleagues' study[13] could have compromised to demonstrate a cause-effect relationship. With regard to antibiotic resistance, the preventive treatment with antibiotics may not be recommendable, although practical and economic advantages were discussed by the industry.[40]

Efficiency of $PGF_{2\alpha}$

$PGF_{2\alpha}$ is a endogenously secreted hormone that causes luteolysis of the corpus luteum[41,42] and causes muscular contraction of various organs including the uterine tract.[43,44] The rationale behind the use of prostaglandins in clinical endometritis is to induce luteolysis of the corpus luteum and to eliminate progesterone production and its immunosuppressive effect.[31] The increase of estrogen levels during the onset of estrus stimulates uterine contractility and clearance of its content and supports the combat against inflammation and infection by triggering influx of neutrophils and immunoglobulins into the uterine mucosa and mucus. In the absence of a corpus luteum, $PGF_{2\alpha}$ increases leukotriene B_4 secretion by the uterus, which supports chemotaxis, cell-mediated cytotoxicity, phagocytosis, and lymphocyte function.[45] $PGF_{2\alpha}$ could stimulate, therefore, uterine involution and reduces the risk for prolonged uterine infection and inflammation in postparturient cows.[46]

For more than 2 decades, $PGF_{2\alpha}$ has been routinely used by veterinarians for the treatment of uterine diseases. It is easy to administer and unexpensive and avoids a potential damage to the uterus associated with intrauterine infusion as well as problems with residues in milk. Over the years and with conflicting reports, many studies have tried to assess the effect of the routine treatment of $PGF_{2\alpha}$ on reproductive performance in a population of postpartum cows with various postpartum conditions. The most common protocols include 2 injections of $PGF_{2\alpha}$ (500 μg cloprostenol IM or 25 mg of dinoprostenol IM) 14 days apart in the second half of the voluntary waiting period as part of a systematic estrus and ovulation synchronization program and as a therapeutic protocol for clinical endometritis. The meta-analysis of Burton and Lean[47] pooled data from 19 reports for a total of 6696 cows to show no effect of $PGF_{2\alpha}$ on the first service pregnancy risk when it was administered on a routine basis to postpartum cows. However, treated cows had significantly less days open than untreated cows.

To assess the effect of $PGF_{2\alpha}$ on cows with clinical endometritis, five clinical trials were included in the present analysis: Two studies[13,24] assessed $PGF_{2\alpha}$ and antibiotic treatment efficiency on clinical endometritis. Leblanc and colleagues[24] showed that administration of at least 2 doses of $PGF_{2\alpha}$ (14 days apart) between 20 and 33 DIM had no benefits on cows with clinical endometritis based on subsequent reproductive performance. Later in postpartum, administration of $PGF_{2\alpha}$ at 35 and 49 DIM in a low- and high-risk group of cows for uterine disease with clinical endometritis, no positive effect was measured.[13] To amplify the potential benefits of $PGF_{2\alpha}$, Hendricks and coworkers[25] administered $PGF_{2\alpha}$ more often and started injections earlier in the postpartum period (2 injections of $PGF_{2\alpha}$ 8 hours apart at 7 and 14 DIM and 1 injection at 22 and 35 DIM with and without Presynch-Ovsynch [3 additional injection of $PGF_{2\alpha}$]) but, again, could not show any significant improvement of the reproductive performance in cows with clinical endometritis compared to untreated animals. Furthermore, the prevalence of clinical endometritis was not changed by all these treatments. No effect of $PGF_{2\alpha}$ was reported in cows with uterine diseases when treated twice, 14 and 28 DIM in a seasonal calving system.[26] In this study, 61% of all cases (n = 180) of postpartum uterine disease were diagnosed as clinical endometritis. Similar results were found with a single $PGF_{2\alpha}$ injection after 21 DIM.[29] A better first service conception risk was measured when $PGF_{2\alpha}$ was given at 42 DIM. However, a very small number (n = 51) of cows was investigated in Feldman and coworkers' trial.

SUMMARY

Implications for Practitioners

From the best scientific evidences available, a single intrauterine infusion of cephapirin benzathine (CB, Metricure) in cows with less than 28 DIM in a seasonal calving system is appropriate to treat clinical endometritis. This therapeutic approach has proved to result in a better reproductive performance compared to untreated cows. There is, however, only weak evidence that CB is as effective to increase reproductive performance in high producing dairy cows with clinical postpartum endometritis in an annual calving system. In contrast to other intrauterine treatments, CB has no side effects or milk withdrawal issues. In addition, other antibiotics, if systemically used or as a intrauterine infusion as a treatment or a preventive approach, did not show any improvement of the uterine condition based on reproductive performance. Similarly, no scientific evidence supports the effectiveness of $PGF_{2\alpha}$ as a treatment for clinical endometritis in postpartum dairy cows.

Implications for Research

Substantial evidence supports the association between clinical endometritis and reduction of subsequent reproductive performance. This relationship exists in seasonal and annual calving systems and therefore with high and low producing dairy cows. Surprisingly, there is still a lack of strong association between the appearance of vaginal discharge and the quantitative assessment of uterine inflammation by cytology[13] and the presence of *A pyogenes*.[8] In addition, variation in susceptibility of *A pyogenes* to antibiotics has been reported.[48] Based on all these observations, it is not surprising that the treatment approach of clinical endometritis is still controversial. More detailed knowledge of the basic physiologic process of uterine involution, the immunologic defense mechanisms of the uterus in postpartum period and the characterization of *A pyogenes* including the mechanisms of its pathogenicity and its susceptibility to antibiotics are needed. In addition, understanding the role of confounders like calving–to–treatment interval and the presence of a functional corpus luteum are critical for a better understanding of the pathophysiology of clinical endometritis in postpartum dairy cows. Since clinical endometritis is a multifactorial disease, a well-planned management protocol is essential for practitioners to develop a global therapeutic and preventive approach for each specific herd.

With the risks of antibiotic resistance in humans, awareness should always be raised on the traditional and empirical use of large-spectrum antibiotics against *A pyogenes*, the most common bacteria involved in the pathogenesis of clinical endometritis in postpartum dairy cows. With the risk of selected resistance, a routine approach may no longer be appropriate. However, the potential availability of new antibiotics with improved bioavailability and the application of new management strategies to prevent clinical endometritis may be promising. With a better understanding of the uterine physiopathology and immune defense, researchers will be able to suggest better diagnostic tools and, eventually, a more efficient therapeutic approach to deal with uterine pathology.

REFERENCES

1. Fourichon C, Seegers H, Malher X. Effect of disease on reproduction in the dairy cow: a meta-analysis. Theriogenology 2000;53:1729–59.
2. Sheldon IM, Lewis GS, LeBlanc S, et al. Defining postpartum uterine disease in cattle. Theriogenology 2006;65:1516–30.
3. Borsberry S, Dobson H. periparturient diseases and their effect on reproductive performance in five dairy herds. Vet Rec 1989;124:217–9.
4. Ferguson J, Galligan D. Assessment of reproductive efficiency in dairy herds. Vet Med Food Anim Compend 2000;22:5150.
5. LeBlanc SJ. Postpartum uterine disease and dairy herd reproductive performance: a review. Vet J 2008;176:102–14.
6. Klucin´ski W, Targowski SP, Winnicka A, et al. Immunological induction of endometritis-model investigations in cows. Zbl Vet MedA 1990;37:148–53.
7. Bondurant R. Inflammation in the bovine female reproductive tract. J Anim Sci 1999;77:101–9.
8. Williams EJ, Fischer DP, Pfeiffer DU, et al. Clinical evaluation of postpartum vaginal mucus reflects uterine bacterial infection and the immune response in cattle. Theriogenology 2005;63:102–17.
9. Galvao KN, Greco LF, Vilela JM, et al. Effect of intrauterine infusion of ceftiofur on uterine health and fertility in dairy cows. J Dairy Sci 2009;92:1532–42.
10. Studer E, Morrow DA. Postpartum evaluation of bovine reproductive potential: comparison of findings from genital tract examination per rectum, uterine culture, and endometrial biopsy. J Am Vet Med Assoc 1978;172:489–94.
11. LeBlanc SJ, Duffield TF, Leslie KE, et al. Defining and diagnosing postpartum clinical endometritis and its impact on reproductive performance in dairy cows. J Dairy Sci 2002;85:2223–36.
12. Kasimanickam R, Duffield TF, Foster RA, et al. A comparison of the cytobrush and uterine lavage techniques to evaluate endometrial cytology in clinically normal postpartum dairy cows. Can Vet J 2005;46:255–9.
13. Dubuc J, Duffield TF, Leslie KE, et al. Randomized clinical trial of antibiotic and prostaglandin treatments for uterine health and reproductive performance in dairy cows. J Dairy Sci 2011;94:1325–38.
14. Runciman DJ, Anderson GA, Malmo J. Comparison of two methods of detecting purulent vaginal discharge in postpartum dairy cows and effect of intrauterine cephapirin on reproductive performance. Aust Vet J 2009;87:369–78.

15. Markusfeld O. Periparturient traits in seven high dairy herds. incidence rates, association with parity, and interrelationships among traits. J Dairy Sci 1987;70:158–66.
16. Guard CL. Costs of clinical disease in dairy cows. Proceedings of Annual Cornell Veterinary Conference, Cornell University. Ithaca (NY), 1994.
17. Wade D, Lewis G. Exogenous prostaglandin F2 alpha stimulates utero-ovarian release of prostaglandin F2 alpha in sheep: a possible component of the luteolytic mechanism of action of exogenous prostaglandin F2 alpha. Domest Anim Endocrinol 1996;13:383–98.
18. Sheldon IM, Cronin J, Goetze L, et al. Defining postpartum uterine disease and the mechanisms of infection and immunity in the female reproductive tract in cattle. Biol Reprod 2009;81:1025–32.
19. Azawi OI. Postpartum uterine infection in cattle. Anim Reprod Sci 2008;105:187–208.
20. Bartlett P, Kirk J, Wilke M, et al. Metritis complex in Michigan Holstein-Friesian cattle: incidence, descriptive epidemiology and estimated economic impact. Prev Vet Med (Netherlands) 1986;4:235–48.
21. Bretzlaff KN. Rationale for treatment of endometritis in the dairy cow. Vet Clin North Am Food Anim Pract 1987;3:593–607.
22. Chalmers TC. A method for assessing the quality of a randomized control trial. Control Clin Trials 1981;2:31–49.
23. Dohmen MJW, Lohuis JACM, Huszenicza GY, et al. The relationship between bacteriological and clinical findings in cows with subacute/chronic endometritis. Theriogenology 1995;43:1379–88.
24. LeBlanc SJ, Duffield TF, Leslie KE, et al. The effect of treatment of clinical endometritis on reproductive performance in dairy cows. J Dairy Sci 2002;85:2237–49.
25. Hendricks KEM, Bartolome JA, Melendez P, et al. Effect of repeated administration of $PGF2\alpha$ in the early post partum period on the prevalence of clinical endometritis and probability of pregnancy at first insemination in lactating dairy cows. Theriogenology 2006;65:1454–64.
26. Glanvill SF, Dobson H. Effect of prostaglandin treatment on the fertility of problem cows. Vet Rec 1991;128:374–6.
27. Runciman DJ, Anderson GA, Malmo J, et al. Efect of intrauterine treatment with cephapirin on the reproductive performance of seasonally calving dairy at risk of endometritis following periparturient disease. Aust Vet J 2008;86:250–8.
28. Thurmond MC, Connor MJ, Picanso JP. Effect of intrauterine antimicrobial treatment in reducing calving-to-conception interval in cows with endometritis. JAVMA 1993; 203:1576–8.
29. Feldman M, Tenhagen G, Emming S, et al. Treatment of chronic bovine endometritis and factors for treatment success. Dtsch Tierrzti Wochenschr 2005;112:10–6.
30. Gautam G, Nakao T, Koike K, et al. Spontaneous recovery or persistence of postpartum endometritis and risk factors for its persistence in Holstein cows. Theriogenology 2010;73:168–79.
31. Lewis GS. Steroidal regulation of uterine resistance to bacterial infection in livestock. Reprod Biol Endocrinol 2003;1:117–21.
32. Herath S, Fisher DP, Werling D, et al. Expression and function of Toll-like receptor 4 in the endometrial cells of the uterus. Endocrinology 2006;147:562–70.
33. Kelton DF, Leslie KE, Etherington WG, et al. Accuracy of rectal palpation and a rapid milk progesterone enzyme immunoassay for determining the presence of a functional corpus luteum in subestrous dairy cows. Can Vet J 1991;32:286–91.
34. Bacalho RC, Galvao KN, Guard CL, et al. Optimizing the accuracy of detecting a functional corpus luteum in dairy cows. Theriogenology 2008;70:199–207.

35. Santos TMA, Caixeta LS, Machado VS, et al. Antimicrobial resistance and presence of virulence factor genes in Arcanobacterium pyogenes isolated from the uterus of postpartum dairy cows. Vet Microbiol 2010;145:84–9.
36. Black WD, Mackay AL Doig PA, et al. A study of drug residues in milk following intrauterine infusion of antibacterial drugs in lactating cows. Can Vet J 1979;20: 354–7.
37. Gilbert RO, Schwark WS. Pharmacologic considerations in the management of peripartum conditions in the cow. Vet Clin North Am Food Anim Pract 1992;8:29–56.
38. Witte TS, Iwersen M, Kaufmann T, et al. Determination of ceftiofur derivatives in serum, endometrial tissue, and lochia in puerperal dairy cows after subcutaneous administration of ceftiofur crystalline free acid. J Dairy Sci 2011;94:284–90.
39. Haggett EF, Wilson WD. Overview of the use of antimicrobials for treatment of bacterial infections in horses. Equine Vet Educ 2008;20:433–48.
40. Galligan D. Economic assessment of animal health performance. Vet Clin North Am Food Anim Pract 2006;22:207–27.
41. Poyser NL. The control of prostaglandin production by the endometrium in relation to luteolysis and menstruation. Prostagland Leukotr Essential Fatty Acids 1995; 53:147–95.
42. Wright PJ, Malmo J. Pharmacologic manipulation of fertility. Vet Clin North Am Food Anim Pract 1992;8:57–89.
43. Hirsbrunner G, Kupfer U, Burkhardt H, et al. The effect of different prostaglandins on intrauterine pressure and uterine motility during diestrus in experimental cows. Theriogenology 1998;50:445–55.
44. Lindell JO, Kindahl H. Exogenous prostaglandin F2α promotes uterine involution in the cow. Acta Vet Scand 1983;24:269–79.
45. Hoedemaker M. Postpartum pathological vaginal discharge: to treat or not to treat. Reprod Dom Anim 1998;33:141–6.
46. Slama H, Vaillancourt D, Goff AK. Leukotriene B4 in cows with normal calving, and in cows with retained fetal membranes and/or uterine subinvolution. Can J Vet Res 1993;57:293–9.
47. Burton NR, Lean IJ. Investigation by meta-analysis of the effect of prostaglandin F2α administered post partum on the reproductive performance of dairy. Vet Rec 1995; 136:90–4.
48. Malinowski E, Lassa H, Markiewicz H, et al. Sensitivity to antibiotics of Arcanobacterium pyogenes and Escherichia coli from the uteri of cows with metritis/endometritis. Vet J 2011;187:234–8.

Evidence-Based Effectiveness of Vaccination Against *Mannheimia haemolytica*, *Pasteurella multocida*, and *Histophilus somni* in Feedlot Cattle for Mitigating the Incidence and Effect of Bovine Respiratory Disease Complex

R.L. Larson, DVM, PhD[a,*], D.L. Step, DVM[b]

KEYWORDS

- Evidence-based • Bovine respiratory disease complex
- *Mannheimia haemolytica* • *Pasteurella multocida*
- *Histophilus somni* • Vaccination

Evidence-based medicine (EBM) was introduced to the medical literature in a 1992 article by the Evidence-based Working Group at McMaster University Health Sciences Centre in Canada to describe the clinical learning strategy they had been developing for over a decade.[1] The principles of EBM are being applied to the veterinary profession under the term "evidence-based veterinary medicine" (EBVM).[2–4] The underlying concepts of EBM and EBVM are rooted in clinical epidemiology and are not new but represent a

The authors have nothing to disclose.
[a] Department of Clinical Sciences, College of Veterinary Medicine, Kansas State University, 1800 Denison Avenue, Manhattan, KS 66506, USA
[b] Department of Veterinary Clinical Sciences, Center for Veterinary Health Sciences, Oklahoma State University, 213 West Farm Road, Stillwater, OK 74078, USA
* Corresponding author.
E-mail address: RLarson@vet.k-state.edu

doi:10.1016/j.cvfa.2011.12.005

formal and explicit effort to increase the occurrence of basing clinical decisions on a dispassionate review of published trials that adequately meet a *priori* standards of experimental design and experimental execution.

Although most clinical decisions in veterinary medicine are based on evidence of some type, some evidence is very strong (rigorously tested in the target species under natural conditions, such as cattle in commercial feedlots in experiments designed to prove a theory to be false), some evidence is very weak (not tested), and some is intermediate.[5–7] The hierarchy of evidence is based on the strength of evidence for causation, the ability of the study to control bias, and the similarity between the study population and the population currently being considered in a clinical setting.

With respect to bacterial vaccination in feedlot cattle, sources regarded as the strongest evidence for the effectiveness of vaccination against *Mannheimia haemolytica*, *Pasteurella multocida,* and *Histophilus somni* for mitigating the incidence and effect of bovine respiratory disease (BRD) complex are randomized controlled clinical trials in feedlot cattle under a typical husbandry environment with adequate blinding of investigators, a clear case-definition of BRD, and adequate intensity and length of follow-up; or systematic reviews of more than 1 trial that meet these criteria. In addition, other available evidence, including studies testing the effects of vaccination of cattle exposed to pathogen-challenged disease models, studies testing the effects of vaccination of cattle in dissimilar production settings (ie, dairy calves), and studies using in vitro methodologies to test vaccination effects can be used as indirect indicators in the clinical decision-making process, particularly when higher levels of evidence are lacking.

The "body of evidence" for this clinical question is the sum of multiple studies investigating the effect of vaccines against *M haemolytica*, *P multocida,* and *H somni* administered to cattle. Each individual research study contributes to that body of evidence and each publication can be ranked on a scale from weak evidence to very strong evidence, which, for the veterinary practitioner, implies an increasing confidence in recommendations based on a particular study. And, although a simple ranking of experimental trial types is helpful to describe ascending levels of evidence, by its simplistic nature, it incorrectly depicts levels of evidence as a one-dimensional and straightforward hierarchy. For example, veterinarians are often confronted with determinations such as—Which is better evidence, a randomized trial in 3 month-old dairy calves (ie, nontarget animals, but a study design with high control of bias and confounding) or a pathogen-challenged disease model study in feedlot cattle (ie, study with less external validity but in the target population)? In these situations, the clinical expertise, experience, and judgment of the veterinarian must be used to aid the ranking of evidence generated by these studies and to guide recommendations for use of bacterial respiratory pathogen vaccines into processing protocols in the field.

Veterinarians considering the strength of evidence must use several perspectives to determine the reliability of research for clinical use.

1. The first consideration is the internal validity of the research, which is determined by the study method and appropriate use of controls for bias. Research reports with good internal validity provide assurance that the results represent an unbiased estimate of the true direction and magnitude of the treatment effect in the study population. For randomized controlled studies, accepted methods of random allocation and blinding of study investigators to the treatment for each experimental unit are key experimental design features to avoid bias and confounding.

2. The second consideration is the population used in the research and its appropriateness as a model for the population that generated the clinical question. Generally, the target species in similar housing and husbandry environments provides stronger evidence than the target species in significantly different housing and husbandry environments, related species, unrelated species, or in vitro methods.
3. And, third, the clinical relevance of the outcomes of the research should be considered with patient- or herd-oriented outcomes (eg, morbidity risk, mortality risk, or average daily weight gain) providing more direct evidence of intervention effectiveness than disease-oriented outcome measurements such as behavior frequency, body temperature, or antibody response.

Using these considerations, the highest rating in all 3 dimensions would provide the highest level of evidence.

MATERIALS AND METHODS

A literature search was conducted to identify studies published in English that reported the effectiveness of *Mannheimia (Pasteurella) haemolytica*, *Pasteurella multocida*, and *Histophilus (Haemophilus) somnus* vaccination in cattle. A search strategy using (*Mannheimia haemolytica* OR *Pasteurella haemolytica* OR *Pasteurella multocida* OR *Haemophilus somnus* OR *Histophilus somni)* AND (respiratory disease OR pneumonia OR pneumonic) AND (bovine OR cattle OR bos) AND (vaccine OR vaccinate) was used to query PubMed (n = 164 references), CAB abstracts (n = 379) and Biologic Abstracts (n = 160) followed by a hand search through cited references (n = 4). A published manuscript is considered a "study" while a "trial" is a direct comparison of a vaccine treatment to a control treatment within a study. A single study may include more than 1 trial. After reading the abstract from each unique publication, 34 studies were included in this review. Fifteen studies (22 trials) were considered the highest level of evidence in that they were trials using feedlot or stocker cattle in North American production settings appropriately allocated to treatment groups with naturally occurring disease.[8–22] One or more trials from 5 other studies were identified that used feedlot cattle in typical North American production settings, but they were weakened by lack of blinding, treatment being confounded by arrival group or other vaccine treatment, or significant loss to follow-up and were discarded from the summary.[23–27] In addition, 3 terminal studies (5 trials) investigated the use of commercially available vaccines in feedlot cattle with a pathogen-challenged disease model[14,28,29]; 3 studies (5 trials) used dairy or beef calves with naturally occurring disease to investigate effects of vaccination[27,30,31]; and 13 studies investigated the use of commercially available vaccines in dairy calves with an induced-disease model.[32–44] Studies were excluded from the review if they did not report original data (primary study); if they did not include a nonvaccinated/placebo control group; if the outcome did not include an assessment of morbidity risk, mortality risk, or extent of lung involvement (eg, only reported serologic titers); or if the same results were published in a more complete form elsewhere. Many studies did not report specific allocation schemes used or whether effective blinding occurred, and some studies used inappropriate statistical tests for the data collected. Studies with obvious limitations due to experimental design were excluded, but studies with poorly described experimental designs were retained.

A meta-analysis was performed, and a Mantel-Haenszel risk ratio (RR) and 95% confidence interval (95% CI) were calculated for each trial reporting cumulative incidence of BRD morbidity or mortality (or crude morbidity or mortality).[45] Calculated

RR less than 1.0 indicates that vaccinates had lower cumulative incidence compared to controls, while RR greater than 1.0 indicates that vaccinates had higher cumulative incidence compared to controls. In order to be considered to have a statistically significantly lower morbidity or mortality cumulative incidence in vaccinates compared to controls, the upper limit of the 95% CI must be below 1.0; while in order to consider the cumulative incidence of morbidity or mortality to be statistically significantly higher in vaccinates compared to controls, the lower limit of the 95% CI must be greater than 1.0. A Forest plot is provided to demonstrate graphically the relative strength of the treatment effects.

RESULTS

Studies Using Feedlot Cattle With Naturally Occurring Disease (Appendix 1)

Data were extracted from the 15 studies (22 trials) that tested the effectiveness of vaccination against 1 or more of the bacterial pathogens *M haemolytica*, *P multocida*, and *H somni* in feedlot cattle for mitigating the incidence and effect of BRD complex using feedlot cattle with naturally occurring disease in order to calculate the RR for each trial (**Appendix 1**). Using the criteria outlined here, these studies are expected to provide the highest level of evidence from the available studies identified in the literature search. A brief account of the studies, including a description of how the cattle were allocated to treatment, the timing of vaccine administration, and a characterization of the vaccines used, can be found in the appendices.

All 22 trials reported a cumulative incidence for morbidity. For some trials the case definition for being considered a case was not specified; other studies had clear case definitions for BRD morbidity. Some studies reported crude morbidity and mortality risk (morbidity or mortality due to any cause), while some studies reported BRD-specific morbidity and mortality risk.

M haemolytica and M haemolytica + P multocida vaccines

Studies investigating the effectiveness of several different commercially available vaccines against *M haemolytica* (15 trials) and *M haemolytica* + *P multocida* (3 trials) were summarized, with 3 of 18 trials reporting a statistically significant reduction in BRD morbidity cumulative incidence in vaccinates compared to controls (eg, upper 95% CI was less than 1.00),[10,16,17] while 4 reported an increased risk of BRD morbidity[8,17,20] and 11[9–15,18–20] reported a decreased risk of BRD morbidity cumulative incidence that was not different from control populations (**Fig. 1**). The summary RR for these trials is 0.93 with a 95% CI that does not cross 1.0 (0.89–0.98), indicating a statistically significant lower risk of morbidity in vaccinated feedlot cattle compared to controls.

The 15 trials that investigated the effect of *M haemolytica*–only vaccine accounted for 90% of the weighted summary RR, and 2 of 15 trials reported a statistically significant reduction in BRD morbidity cumulative incidence in vaccinates compared to controls,[16,17] while 3 reported an increased risk of BRD morbidity[17,20] and 10[9–15,18–20] reported a decreased risk of BRD morbidity cumulative incidence that was not different from controls. The 3 trials that investigated the effect of *M haemolytica* + *P multocida* vaccination accounted for 10% of the weighted summary RR. One of the 3 trials reported a statistically significant reduction in BRD morbidity cumulative incidence in vaccinates compared to controls,[23] while 1 reported an increased risk of BRD morbidity[8] and 1 reported a decreased risk of BRD morbidity cumulative incidence that was not different from control populations.[23]

Evaluating mortality RR in 9 studies that measured BRD-specific or crude mortality risk indicates that 7 trials reported decreased cumulative mortality incidence that was

Study or Subgroup	Vaccinated Events	Vaccinated Total	Control Events	Control Total	Weight	Risk Ratio M-H, Random, 95% CI
Amstutz a 1981	38	108	33	107	1.4%	1.14 [0.78, 1.67]
Bateman 1988	29	90	32	86	1.3%	0.87 [0.58, 1.30]
Bechtol 1996	100	295	124	296	4.3%	0.81 [0.66, 1.00]
Bechtol 1996	78	161	91	160	4.3%	0.85 [0.69, 1.05]
Frank 2002	37	60	39	60	2.7%	0.95 [0.72, 1.25]
Ives 1999	60	162	75	162	2.9%	0.80 [0.62, 1.04]
Jim 1988	444	781	766	1291	17.2%	0.96 [0.89, 1.03]
Loan 1989	3	50	10	50	0.1%	0.30 [0.09, 1.03]
MacGregor 2003	447	1652	480	1652	11.6%	0.93 [0.83, 1.04]
Malcolm-Callis 1994	16	60	28	59	0.9%	0.56 [0.34, 0.92]
McLean a 1990	89	147	109	152	6.4%	0.84 [0.72, 1.00]
McLean b 1990	116	160	109	152	8.4%	1.01 [0.88, 1.16]
Purdy 1986	34	41	52	59	6.2%	0.94 [0.80, 1.11]
Smith 1986	55	218	73	223	2.3%	0.77 [0.57, 1.04]
Thorlakson a 1990	122	284	122	289	5.1%	1.02 [0.84, 1.23]
Thorlakson b 1990	134	291	122	289	5.4%	1.09 [0.91, 1.31]
Thorlakson c 1990	107	276	122	289	4.6%	0.92 [0.75, 1.12]
Thorlakson d 1990	259	363	274	368	14.8%	0.96 [0.88, 1.05]
Total (95% CI)		**5199**		**5744**	**100.0%**	**0.93 [0.89, 0.98]**
Total events	2168		2661			

Heterogeneity: Tau² = 0.00; Chi² = 21.23, df = 17 (P = 0.22); I² = 20%
Test for overall effect: Z = 2.97 (P = 0.003)

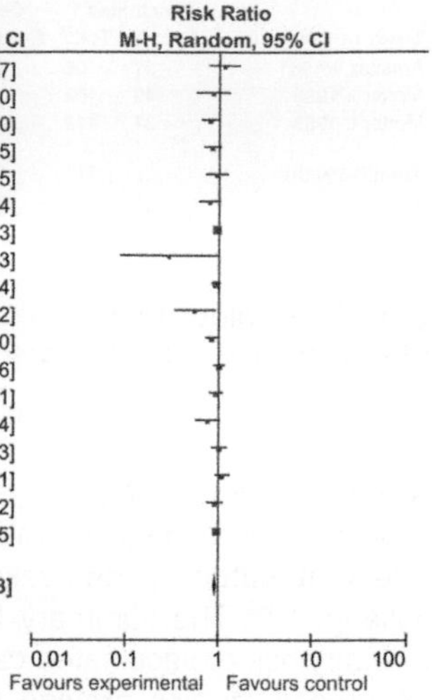

Fig. 1. Forest plot of RR for 18 trials comparing cumulative morbidity incidence of feedlot cattle vaccinated against *M haemolytica* (15 trials) or *M haemolytica* + *P multocida* (3 trials) compared to controls.

not different in vaccinates relative to controls, while 2 reported an increased risk of mortality that was not different from control populations.[10,12,15–18,20] An additional 6 trials reported cumulative mortality incidence, but the RR could not be calculated because of nonevents (zero for very low count cells) (**Fig. 2**). The summary RR for these trials is 0.76 with a 95% CI that crosses 1.0 (0.56–1.04), indicating mortality risk in vaccinated feedlot cattle is not statistically different than that of controls.

M haemolytica + H somni vaccine studies

One study investigated the effectiveness of a commercially available vaccine against *M haemolytica* + *H somni* in feedlot cattle with natural disease challenge.[21] In this study, vaccinated cattle had statistically significantly lower morbidity compared to controls. There were no deaths in the vaccinates or controls (**Appendix 1**).

Study or Subgroup	Vaccinated Events	Vaccinated Total	Control Events	Control Total	Weight	Risk Ratio M-H, Random, 95% CI
Bechtol 1996	5	295	4	296	5.8%	1.25 [0.34, 4.62]
Bechtol 1996	2	161	2	160	2.6%	0.99 [0.14, 6.97]
Ives 1999	6	162	10	162	10.1%	0.60 [0.22, 1.61]
MacGregor 2003	22	1652	31	1652	33.7%	0.71 [0.41, 1.22]
Malcolm-Callis 1986	1	60	3	59	2.0%	0.33 [0.04, 3.06]
McLean a 1990	7	147	11	152	11.7%	0.66 [0.26, 1.65]
McLean b 1990	14	160	11	152	17.2%	1.21 [0.57, 2.58]
Purdy 1986	2	41	6	59	4.1%	0.48 [0.10, 2.26]
Thorlakson d 1990	8	363	12	368	12.7%	0.68 [0.28, 1.63]
Total (95% CI)		**3041**		**3060**	**100.0%**	**0.76 [0.56, 1.04]**
Total events	67		90			

Heterogeneity: Tau² = 0.00; Chi² = 3.41, df = 8 (P = 0.91); I² = 0%
Test for overall effect: Z = 1.70 (P = 0.09)

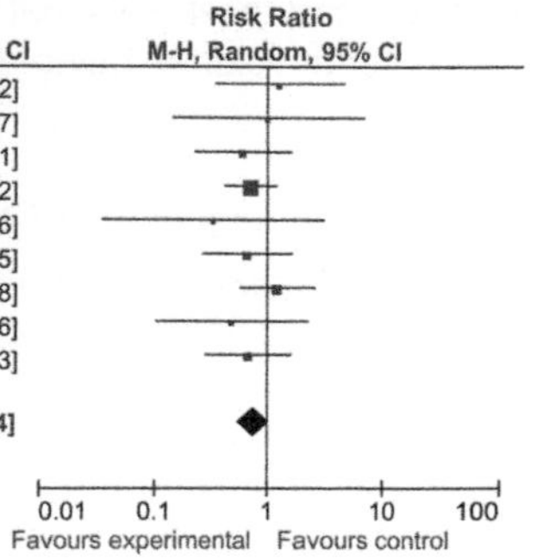

Fig. 2. Forest plot of RR for 9 trials comparing cumulative mortality incidence of feedlot cattle vaccinated against *M haemolytica* (7 trials) or *M haemolytica* + *P multocida* (2 trials) compared to controls.

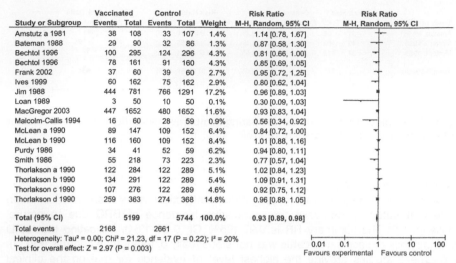

Study or Subgroup	Vaccinated Events	Vaccinated Total	Control Events	Control Total	Weight	Risk Ratio M-H, Random, 95% CI
Amstutz a 1981	21	106	33	107	30.4%	0.64 [0.40, 1.03]
Morter a 1983	49	102	34	102	36.1%	1.44 [1.03, 2.03]
Morter b 1983	31	102	34	102	33.5%	0.91 [0.61, 1.36]
Total (95% CI)		**310**		**311**	**100.0%**	**0.97 [0.61, 1.54]**
Total events	101		101			

Heterogeneity: Tau² = 0.12; Chi² = 7.92, df = 2 (P = 0.02); I² = 75%

Test for overall effect: Z = 0.14 (P = 0.89)

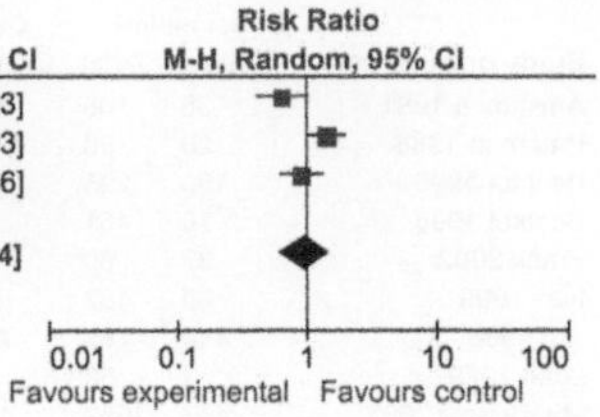

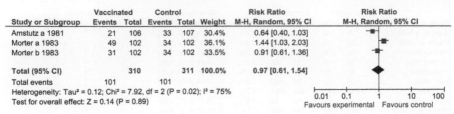

Fig. 3. Forest plot of RR for 3 trials comparing cumulative morbidity incidence of feedlot cattle vaccinated against *H somni* to controls.

H somni vaccine studies

Three trials were identified that investigated the effectiveness of *H somni* vaccination of feedlot cattle to decrease the cumulative incidence of BRD due to natural challenge.[8,22] The summary RR is 0.97 (95% CI, 0.61–1.54), indicating that BRD morbidity risk of vaccinated cattle was not statistically different than controls (**Fig. 3**).

As these studies provide the highest level of evidence for making the clinical decision about the effectiveness of vaccination against the pathogens *M haemolytica*, *P multocida,* and *H somni* in feedlot cattle for mitigating the incidence and effect of BRD complex, the weight of evidence from these 22 trials is particularly important. The summary RR indicates that these studies indicate that vaccination against *M haemolytica* or *M haemolytica* + *P multocida* has the potential to decrease the incidence of BRD complex in feedlot cattle, but the numerical decrease in mortality risk was not statistically different from controls. Much less evidence is available to determine the effectiveness of vaccination against *H somni* in feedlot cattle, and although these studies using natural disease challenge indicate that the risk of BRD does not appear to be affected by vaccination against this pathogen, we have very little power to detect a true difference if it did exist.

Studies Using Feedlot Cattle With Pathogen-Challenged Disease Models (Appendix 2)

M haemolytica vaccines

Three studies reporting 5 trials were identified that used feedlot cattle to evaluate the association between vaccination with commercially available *M haemolytica* vaccines and mortality risk and lung lesion severity following induced disease with a transthoracic inoculation of *M haemolytica*.[14,28,29] All 5 trials reported increased survival post challenge, and the 4 trials that reported lung severity indicated decreased percentage of total lung volume being classified as pneumonic in vaccinates compared to controls.

Studies Using Dairy or Beef Calves With Naturally Occurring Disease (Appendix 3)

M haemolytica and M haemolytica + P multocida vaccines

Studies using dairy or beef calves during the first 3 to 6 months of life to test the efficacy of a vaccine against *M haemolytica* or a combination vaccine against *M haemolytica* + *P multocida* are not considered to provide a high level of evidence for clinical questions arising from feedlot cattle health problems because of differences in age, housing, and management. **Figure 4** depicts the Forest plots of the RR for BRD morbidity for 3 trials using dairy calves vaccinated against *M haemolytica* (2 trials) or *M haemolytica* + *P multocida* (1 trial).[27,30] **Figure 5** depicts the Forest plot of the RR for crude mortality for 2 dairy calf trials evaluating *M haemolytica* vaccine.[27]

Study or Subgroup	Experimental Events	Experimental Total	Control Events	Control Total	Weight	Risk Ratio M-H, Random, 95% CI
Aubry 2001	32	179	32	179	25.6%	1.00 [0.64, 1.56]
Smith 1985a	31	73	59	77	36.6%	0.55 [0.41, 0.74]
Smith 1985b	34	74	58	78	37.8%	0.62 [0.47, 0.82]
Total (95% CI)		**326**		**334**	**100.0%**	**0.67 [0.49, 0.91]**
Total events	97		149			

Heterogeneity: Tau² = 0.04; Chi² = 5.15, df = 2 (P = 0.08); I² = 61%
Test for overall effect: Z = 2.54 (P = 0.01)

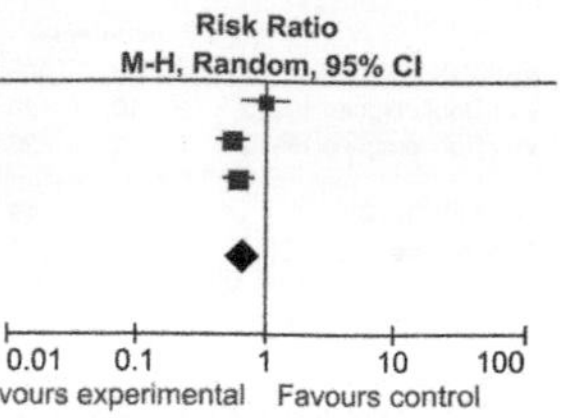

Fig. 4. Forest plot of RR for 3 trials comparing cumulative morbidity incidence of dairy calves vaccinated against *M haemolytica* or *M haemolytica* + *P multocida* compared to controls.

The trials that evaluated the effectiveness of *M haemolytica* or *M haemolytica* + *P multocida* revealed summary RR indicating a statistically significant reduction in BRD morbidity (**Fig. 4**), but not crude mortality (**Fig. 5**) in vaccinated calves compared to controls.

M haemolytica + *H somni* vaccine studies

Calves vaccinated with a genetically attenuated leukotoxin of *M haemolytica* combined with bacterial extracts of *M haemolytica* and *H somni* did not have statistically significantly different risk of BRD morbidity compared to controls (**Fig. 6**).[31]

SUMMARY

The clinical question of whether to use commercially available vaccines against bacterial pathogens associated with BRD in feedlot cattle is important to the veterinarians and producers making the decision, as well as to the health and well-being of feedlot cattle. Making an evidence-based clinical decision based primarily on published, scientifically accepted controlled trials using feedlot cattle, with supportive information from published trials using pathogen-challenged disease models or using dairy or beef calves housed and managed under different husbandry systems, requires not only the gathering and summarizing of the available information but also considering the context of specific clinical questions.

The summary data would indicate potential benefit for vaccination of feedlot cattle against *M haemolytica* and *P multocida* with no evidence of benefit for vaccination against *H somni* for mitigating the incidence and effect of BRD complex. Unfortunately, the published body of evidence does not provide a consistent estimate of the direction and magnitude of effectiveness in feedlot cattle vaccination against *M haemolytica, P multocida*, or *H somni*.

One limitation for the conclusions that can be drawn from this group of studies includes the fact that all the feedlot studies with natural disease challenge mixed

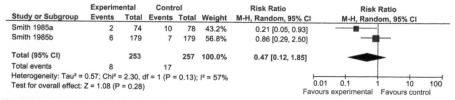

Study or Subgroup	Experimental Events	Experimental Total	Control Events	Control Total	Weight	Risk Ratio M-H, Random, 95% CI
Smith 1985a	2	74	10	78	43.2%	0.21 [0.05, 0.93]
Smith 1985b	6	179	7	179	56.8%	0.86 [0.29, 2.50]
Total (95% CI)		**253**		**257**	**100.0%**	**0.47 [0.12, 1.85]**
Total events	8		17			

Heterogeneity: Tau² = 0.57; Chi² = 2.30, df = 1 (P = 0.13); I² = 57%
Test for overall effect: Z = 1.08 (P = 0.28)

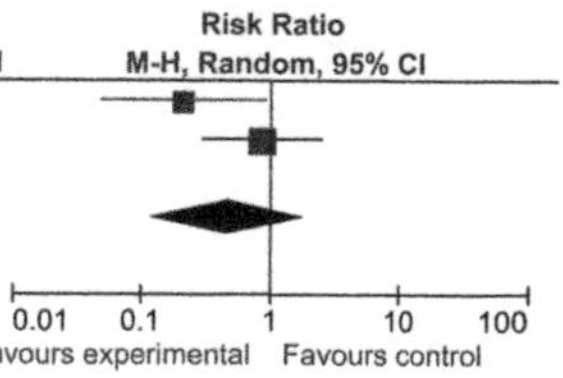

Fig. 5. Forest plot of RR for 2 trials comparing cumulative mortality incidence of dairy calves vaccinated against *M haemolytica* compared to controls.

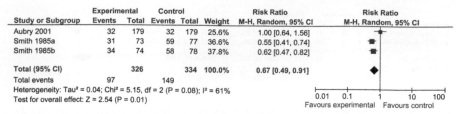

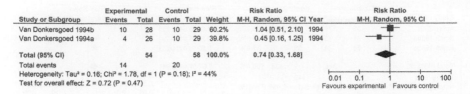

Study or Subgroup	Experimental Events	Experimental Total	Control Events	Control Total	Weight	Risk Ratio M-H, Random, 95% CI	Year
Van Donkersgoed 1994b	10	28	10	29	60.2%	1.04 [0.51, 2.10]	1994
Van Donkersgoed 1994a	4	26	10	29	39.8%	0.45 [0.16, 1.25]	1994
Total (95% CI)		**54**		**58**	**100.0%**	**0.74 [0.33, 1.68]**	
Total events	14		20				

Heterogeneity: $Tau^2 = 0.16$; $Chi^2 = 1.78$, df = 1 (P = 0.18); $I^2 = 44\%$
Test for overall effect: Z = 0.72 (P = 0.47)

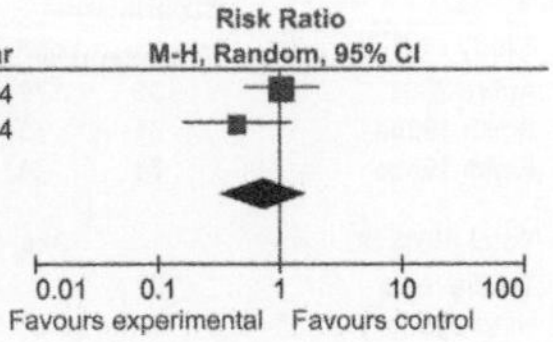

Fig. 6. Forest plot of RR for 2 trials comparing cumulative morbidity incidence of dairy calves vaccinated against *M haemolytica* + *H somni* compared to controls.

vaccinated and unvaccinated calves in the same feedlot pens. This mixing may underestimate the value of vaccination because of the phenomena of herd immunity. In mixed pens, the vaccinated calves may reduce the disease challenge for unvaccinated controls and unvaccinated calves may increase the disease challenge for vaccinated calves compared to the exposure expected when entire pens are either vaccinated or not vaccinated. Another limitation is that some studies reported crude morbidity and mortality while other studies reported BRD-specific morbidity and mortality. Approximately 59% of the weighted summary RR for morbidity in the feedlot studies was derived from studies using a case definition for BRD as the criteria for being classified as a morbid animal, while 41% of the weighted summary RR came from studies reporting the effect of vaccination in all causes of morbidity. Similarly, approximately 57% of the weighted summary RR for mortality in the feedlot studies came from studies specifying mortalities associated with BRD, while 43% of the weighted summary RR was derived from studies reporting the effect of vaccination on all causes of mortality. If non-BRD mortalities were evenly distributed between vaccinates and controls in these studies, aggregating mortality of all causes to test the association with vaccination status will decrease the RR between vaccinates and nonvaccinated controls.

A thorough search of the published literature and a structured meta-analysis to produce a summary Mantel-Haenszel RR and 95% CI are helpful tools for making an assessment of the evidence for the effectiveness of vaccination against *M haemolytica*, *P multocida,* and *H somni* for mitigating the incidence and effect of BRD complex in feedlot cattle. However, because of the limitations of the studies used in the meta-analysis and the various specific clinical situations that feedlot veterinarians and producers confront, it is necessary to combine this summary with other sources of information and unpublished data, as well as continued monitoring of recommendations to arrive at the best advice for feedlot clients.

REFERENCES

1. Evidence-Based Medicine Working Group. Evidence-based medicine: a new approach to teaching the practice of medicine. JAMA 1992;268:2420–5.
2. Keene BW. Towards evidence-based veterinary medicine [editorial]. J Vet Intern Med 2000;14:118–9.
3. Doig GS. Evidence-based veterinary medicine: what it is, what it isn't and how to do it. Aust Vet J 2003;81:412–5.
4. Roudebush P, Allen TA, Dodd CE, et al. Evidence-based medicine: applications to veterinary clinical nutrition. J Am Vet Med Assoc 2004;224:1766–71.
5. Sackett DL. Rules of evidence and clinical recommendations. Can J Cardiol 1993;9:487–9.
6. Dans AL, Dans LF, Guyatt GH, et al. Users' guide to the medical literature. XIV. How to decide on the applicability of clinical trial results to your patient. JAMA 1998;279:545–9.

7. Berg AO. Dimensions of evidence. In: Geyman JP, Deyo RA, Ramsey SD, editors: Evidence-based clinical practice: concepts and approaches. Boston: Butterworth-Heinemann; 2000.
8. Amstutz HE, Horstman LA, Morter RL. Clinical evaluation of the efficacy of *Haemophilus somnus* and *Pasteurella* sp. bacterins. Bov Pract 1981;16:106–8.
9. Bateman KG. Efficacy of a *Pasteurella haemolytica* vaccine/bacterial extract in the prevention of bovine respiratory disease in recently shipped feedlot calves. Can Vet J 1988;29:838–9.
10. Bechtol DT, Jones GF. Can a Pasteurella vaccine prevent respiratory disease in calves in a backgrounding lot? Vet Med 1996;91:1042–5.
11. Frank GH, Briggs RE, Duff GC, et al. Effects of vaccination prior to transit and administration of florfenicol at time of arrival in a feedlot on the health of transported calves and detection of *Mannheimia haemolytica* in nasal secretions. Am J Vet Res 2002;63:251–6.
12. Ives S, Drouillard J, Anderson D, et al. Comparison of morbidity and performance among stressed feeder calves following vaccination with PYRAMID MLV 4 or PYRAMID 4 + PRESPONSE SQ. Kansas State University, Cattlemen's Day, Report of Progress 1999;831:126–9.
13. Jim K, Guichon T, Shaw G. Protecting feedlot calves from pneumonic pasteurellosis. Vet Med 1988;83:1084–7.
14. Loan RW, Tigges MG, Purdy CW. A tissue culture-derived *Pasteurella haemolytica* vaccine. Bov Pract 1989;24:22–4.
15. MacGregor S, Smith D, Perino LJ, et al. An evaluation of the effectiveness of a commercial *Mannheimia* (*Pasteurella*) *haemolytica* vaccine in a commercial feedlot. Bov Pract 2003;37:78–82.
16. Malcolm-Callis KJ, Galyean ML, Duff GC. Effects of dietary supplemental protein source and a *Pasteurella haemolytica* toxoid on performance and health of newly received calves. Agri Pract 1994;15:22–8.
17. McLean GS, Smith RA, Gill RA, et al. An evaluation of an inactivated, leukotoxin-rich, cell-free *Pasteurella haemolytica* vaccine for prevention of undifferentiated bovine respiratory disease. Okla State Univ Anim Sci Res Rep MP-129 1990:135–40.
18. Purdy CW, Livingston CW, Frank GH, et al. A live *Pasteurella haemolytica* vaccine efficacy trial. J Am Vet Med Assoc 1986;188:589–91.
19. Smith RA, Gill DR, Hicks RB. Improving the performance of stocker and feedlot calves with a live *Pasteurella haemolytica* vaccine. Vet Med 1986;81:978–81.
20. Thorlakson B, Martin W, Peters D. A field trial to evaluate the efficacy of a commercial *Pasteurella haemolytica* bacterial extract in preventing bovine respiratory disease. Can Vet J 1990;31:573–9.
21. Van Donkersgoed J, Schumann FJ, Harland RJ, et al. The effect of route and dosage of immunization on the serological response to a *Pasteurella haemolytica* and *Haemophilus somnus vaccine* in feedlot calves. Can Vet J 1993;34:731–5.
22. Morter RL, Amstutz HE. Evaluating the efficacy of a *Haemophilus somnus* bacterin in a controlled field trial. Bov Pract 1983;18:82–3.
23. Bechtol DT, Ballinger RT, Sharp AJ. Field trial of a *Pasteurella haemolytica* toxoid administered at spring branding and in the feedlot. Agri-Pract 1991;12:6–14.
24. Bennett BW. Efficacy of Pasteurella bacterins for yearling feedlot cattle. Bov Pract 1982;3:26–30.
25. Martin W, Acres S, Janzen E, et al. A field trial of preshipment vaccination of calves. Can Vet J 1984;25:145–7.
26. Ribble CS, Jim GK, Janzen ED. Efficacy of immunization of feedlot calves with a commercial *Haemophilus somnus* bacterin. Can J Vet Res 1988;52:191–8.

27. Smith CK, Davidson JN, Henry CW Jr. Evaluating a live vaccine for *Pasteurella haemolytica* in dairy calves. Vet Med 1985;80:78–88.
28. Confer AW, Fulton RW. Evaluation of *Pasteurella* and *Haemophilus* vaccines. Proc 27th Conv AABP. Pittsburgh (PA):American Association of Bovine Practitioners; 1995. p. 136–41.
29. Confer AW, Ayalew S, Panciera RJ, et al. Immunogenicity of recombinant *Mannheimia haemolytica* serotype 1 outer membrane protein PlpE and augmentation of a commercial vaccine. Vaccine 2003;21/22:2821–9.
30. Aubry P, Warnick LD, Guard CL, et al. Health and performance of young dairy calves vaccinated with a modified-live *Mannheimia haemolytica* and *Pasteurella multocida* vaccine. J Am Vet Med Assoc 2001;219:1739–42.
31. Van Donkersgoed J, Potter AA, Mollison B, et al. The effect of a combined *Pasteurella haemolytica* and *Haemophilus somnus* vaccine and a modified-live bovine respiratory syncytial virus vaccine against enzootic pneumonia in young beef calves. Can Vet J 1994;35:239–41.
32. Blanchard-Channell MT, Ashfaq MK, Kadel WL. Efficacy of streptomycin-dependent, live *Pasteurella haemolytica* vaccine against challenge exposure to *Pasteurella haemolytica* in cattle. Am J Vet Res 1987;48:637–42.
33. Cardella MA, Adviento MA, Nervig RM. Vaccination studies against experimental bovine Pasteurella pneumonia. Can J Vet Res 1987;51:204–11.
34. Catt DM, Chengappa MM, Kadel WL, et al. Preliminary studies with a live streptomycin-dependent *Pasteurella multocida* and *Pasteurella haemolytica* vaccine for the prevention of bovine pneumonic pasteurellosis. Can J Comp Med 1985;49:366–71.
35. Chengappa MM, McLaughlin BG, Craft DL. Bovine pneumonic pasteurellosis: efficacy testing a live vaccine. Vet Med 1998;83:837–40.
36. Conlon JAR, Gallo GF, Shewen PE, et al. Comparison of protection of experimentally challenged cattle vaccinated once or twice with a *Pasteurella haemolytica* bacterial extract vaccine. Can J Vet Res 1995;59:179–82.
37. DeBey BM, Roth JA, Brogden KA, et al. *In vitro* lymphocyte proliferative responses and gamma-interferon production as measures of cell-mediated immunity of cattle exposed to *Pasteurella haemolytica*. Can J Vet Res 1996;60:263–70.
38. Shewen PE, Wilkie BN. Vaccination of calves with leukotoxic culture supernatant from *Pasteurella haemolytica*. Can J Vet Res 1988;52:30–6.
39. Shewen PE, Lee CW, Perets A, et al. Efficacy of recombinant sialoglycoprotease in protection of cattle against pneumonic challenge with *Mannheimia (Pasteurella) haemolytica* A1. Vaccine 2003;21:1901–6.
40. Shewen PE, Sharp A, Wilkie BN. Efficacy testing a *Pasteurella haemolytica* extract vaccine. Vet Med 1988;83:1078–83.
41. Srinand S, Mahewsaran SK, Amees TR, et al. Evaluation of efficacy of three commercial vaccines against experimental bovine pneumonic pasteurellosis. Vet Microsc 1996;52:81–9.
42. Berghaus LJ, Corbeil LB, Berghaus RD, et al. Effects of dual vaccination for bovine respiratory syncytial virus and *Haemophilus somnus* on immune responses. Vaccine 2006;24:6018–27.
43. Cairns R, Chu HJ, Chavez LG, et al. Efficacy of an outer membrane complex *Haemophilus somnus* bacterin in preventing symptoms following *Haemophilus somnus* challenge. Agri-Pract 1993;14:35–7.
44. Groom SC, Little PB. Effects of vaccination of calves against induced *Haemophilus somnus* pneumonia. Am J Vet Res 1988;49:793–800.
45. Review Manager (RevMan), Version 5.1. Copenhagen: The Nordic Cochrane Centre, The Cochrane Collaboration, 2011.

Overview of Meta-Analysis of Monensin in Dairy Cattle

Todd F. Duffield, DVM, DVSc[a,*], Ahmad Rabiee, DVM, PhD[b],
Ian J. Lean, BVSc, PhD, MACVSc[b]

KEYWORDS

• Meta-analysis • Monensin • Metabolic • Production
• Health • Dairy

Meta-analyses represent a particularly useful subset of quantitative, systematic literature review. These provide the highest levels of evidence in medicine. Only large, randomized multicenter clinical trials approach these for strength of evidence. Meta-analysis is a powerful analytic method used to quantify the impact of an intervention across several trials. It is important to note, however, that no single study is more powerful than the meta-analysis of well-conducted studies to which that study contributes. Meta-analysis is a quantitative method that complements a systematic review process.

Advantages of meta-analysis over a qualitative review include the opportunity to produce a quantitative, weighted estimate of the effect of an intervention. This approach avoids the traditional literature review of an intervention in which studies are accorded equal value or a perceived value based on quality criteria considered important by the reviewer. One of the results of meta-analysis is a pooled weighted estimate of effect of intervention; others are weighted mean responses, an assessment of the consistency of response (heterogeneity) and the opportunity to explore causes of variation in responses. This heterogeneity can be explored by means of meta-regression and subpopulation analysis that allow significant effects to be quantified and better identify where an intervention will be most effective. This is an emerging field and represents an important, underused tool of veterinary medicine. This article will discuss the merits and methods of meta-analysis, primarily using a recently published series of articles that assessed the impact of monensin in lactating dairy cattle. Full details of these studies can be found in Duffield and colleagues.[3–5]

This work was partially supported by a research grant from Elanco Animal Health.
The authors have nothing to disclose.
[a] Department of Population Medicine, Ontario Veterinary College, University of Guelph, Guelph, ON, Canada, N1G 2W1
[b] SBScibus, 2 Broughton Street, Camden, NSW 2570, Australia
* Corresponding author.
E-mail address: tduffiel@uoguelph.ca

Vet Clin Food Anim 28 (2012) 107–119
doi:10.1016/j.cvfa.2011.12.009 vetfood.theclinics.com
0749-0720/12/$ – see front matter

PROBLEMS AND OBJECTIVES FOR META-ANALYSIS OF MONENSIN IN DAIRY CATTLE

Although double-blind randomized clinical trials are excellent sources of results for making evidence-based decisions, a frustration for some studies, at least, is that there is a variable response in outcome. Simply put, there are studies where a product may have worked and others where the product did not work. Studies can be consistent in the direction of effect, but be of very different magnitude, but in some cases the direction of the effect can differ. Salesman would like to highlight those studies where the product worked and deemphasize those where it did not work. The difficult question for the end user is: will it work in the situation that I intend to use it or to recommend it in?

There are 2 primary reasons for heterogeneity—clinical heterogeneity and methodologic diversity—and these, along with underlying chance distributions, result in statistical heterogeneity.

Clinical Heterogeneity

Reasons for this heterogeneity might include differences in populations of animals on which studies were conducted (demographics such as age, breed, production level), differences in physiologic state (whether lactating, stage of lactation, whether pregnant, etc), regional differences in management of animals, and dietary differences. The outcomes measured may also subtly differ or even markedly differ.

Methodologic Diversity

This includes type of intervention used (in this case, there were different formulations of monensin), dose of intervention, and concurrent interventions or diets. In the case of the monensin study, all these varied.

Statistical Heterogeneity

While statistical heterogeneity is primarily a function of clinical and methodologic heterogeneity, the underlying chance distributions of results will also contribute to heterogeneity and interventions such as monensin, which have small, but potentially important effects, will, on occasions, produce small negative results simply due to the distribution of responses around the true effect.

BACKGROUND OF MONENSIN IN DAIRY CATTLE

Monensin was identified as a very suitable topic for meta-analytical evaluation. We were aware that there was a large number of studies of this intervention and that there was some controversy over responses to the intervention. There were several questions that arose in regard to the predicted responses to monensin in dairy cattle. Some studies existed in which there was variation in the direction of effect—for example, milk production did not increase significantly[6]; other studies demonstrated that monensin decreased milk fat percentage[7]; whereas other studies did not find that effect.[8,9] Similarly, the effect of monensin on serum glucose was reported to vary in direction, with some studies demonstrating increases in serum glucose[10] and others not[11] and still others showing decreases.[12] There appeared to be very confusing responses in retained placenta and calving difficulty with studies that approached significance in either direction.

A very good traditional literature review by Ipharragure and Clark had been published just before we undertook the meta-analysis.[13] The review provided estimates for some outcomes including milk production effects of monensin. These reviews of literature are useful; however, traditional reviews weight all studies equally and do not account for sample size or variance differences between studies. More importantly, these types of summaries do not provide evidence or reasons for heterogeneity of response.

The main objectives for conducting a meta-analysis of monensin effects in lactating dairy cattle were to summarize the literature on impacts of monensin on:

1. Serum/blood metabolites
2. Milk production parameters (including dry matter intake [DMI], yield, efficiency, and components)
3. Health and reproductive performance.

LITERATURE REVIEW—SCOPE: UNPUBLISHED AND PUBLISHED DATA, EXCLUSION CRITERIA, DATA EXTRACTION

This project addressed the literature from the 3 perspectives of responses of blood metabolites, milk and milk components production and concentration, and health and reproduction. A broad literature search in 2007 was conducted using several search engines (Google Scholar, Agricola, PubMed) and the following key words (monensin or Rumensin and dairy and cow). In addition, Elanco Animal Health (manufacturers of Rumensin) was contacted for information on unpublished studies. They provided contact information for researchers or raw data from studies. The intention of attempting to gather both published and unpublished data is to reduce publication bias (to be discussed later). The necessary constraint to this strategy is to ensure that the inclusion and exclusion criteria for studies are standardized.

A priori criteria were constructed to screen articles for suitability into the meta-analysis database. If these criteria are constructed to be too restrictive, the meta-analysis becomes narrow in scope. However, criteria that are too liberal increase the probability that the quality of the data will be lower. In a study of the effect of organic minerals on cattle, Rabiee and coworkers found the following differences in published and unpublished manuscripts. [14] It is clear that there is a difference in quality of articles that were published in this case **Table 1**.

The following criteria were required for inclusion of a study into the meta-analysis: randomization of treatments, use of an appropriate control group, and a reported measure of dispersion. If there was no indication in the article that treatments were assigned randomly, then that article or study was rejected. Randomization of treatments can be managed in a number of ways; the critical factor is that there is no evidence of bias in the assignment of treatments. Blinding of treatments so that the researchers cannot identify the actual treatment and placebo further strengthens this, but blinding was not a requirement for this project because it would have eliminated too many articles. This finding has been consistent in all meta-analyses conducted by the authors. Consequently, there is a need for improved conduct of studies in regard to both formal randomization and blinding of studies in the veterinary and animal science literature.

Use of an appropriate control group means that there was either an untreated or a placebo-treated control to compare to monensin. Some studies compared one treatment to another treatment and these were rejected since the objective was to compare the effect of monensin to cows not being treated. Studies that reported standard errors, standard deviations, or *P* values where measures of dispersion could be estimated were included. However, there were some articles where these were not reported and the article was rejected, or the measure of variance was estimated using the probability, number of animals in each group, and the differences in the effects between groups using a *t* distribution (Sanchez and colleagues, 2004).[15] In a few cases, some outcomes within an article had measures of dispersion reported, but others did not. In these cases, the authors were contacted to enquire about the possibility of obtaining these data and this was a successful approach in some (3) cases.

We also elected to reject articles that were of a Latin square design and also any articles that involved an acidosis challenge. Obviously, acidosis challenge models serve a purpose for scientific study, but these were not suitable for inclusion in our meta-analysis, since we were trying to estimate benefits of monensin for use on typical farms and most farms would not have continuous acidosis challenges. In other words, the acidosis challenge models were artificial and did not represent normal industry practices. The Latin square designs posed a different problem. Each cow has multiple, replicated treatments, and the error structure of these studies ensures that it is much more difficult to extract appropriate measures of dispersion to compare these treatments with the other studies. The second concern with Latin squares is the possibility of treatment carryover effects—specifically, the possibility that nutrients accreted in one treatment period could be mobilized in another, thereby confounding responses to treatment. Further, changes in rumen function triggered by a particular treatment may extend for a prolonged period and there was evidence of variation in the washout times used between treatment periods to account for this problem.

Any article included also needed to have evaluated at least 1 of the 3 areas of interest. Consequently, a number of excellent articles were rejected because the outcomes did not address the key areas on interest. Articles rejected for lack of immediate relevance included studies on neutrophil function and Johne's disease. Finally, 59 (74%) articles from 80 eligible studies evaluated provided useable data and appropriate measures of variance on the selected variable outcomes.

Once the articles were selected, the data were extracted. For each outcome, the number of cows (N), mean, and standard error (or estimate) were extracted. For the dichotomous data, numbers of cattle in groups were extracted, and for reproductive data, the raw data for a number of the studies were obtained. Other data that could be potentially useful to explain heterogeneity, if present, were also extracted. These additional data included variables such as dose and method of delivery of monensin—topdress, total mixed ration (TMR), controlled release capsule (CRC)—stage of lactation at treatment start, duration of the study, feed information if presented, and other relevant findings.

DATA ANALYSIS AND REPORTING: SUMMARY STATISTICS, FOREST PLOT, HETEROGENEITY

The meta-analysis was conducted on the extracted outcomes using Stata (Intercooled Stata V. 9.0; StataCorp, College Station, TX, USA) and random effects models. The effect size estimate analysis was conducted using a standardized z statistic; however, for all significant outcomes, the unit of measurement was converted to the International System of Units (S.I.) values to allow the calculation of weighted mean differences of treatment relative to control. This included the conversion of all urea-N values in mg/dL to urea in mmol/L by multiplying the urea-N value by 0.357.

The χ^2 test for heterogeneity[1] was used to assess the amount of variation in experiment level effect size. In addition, the heterogeneity of results among trials was quantified using the I^2 statistic.[2] This measure is also called an uncertainty interval and is measured in values between 0% and 100%. An I^2 value greater than 50% is considered to have substantial heterogeneity.

Table 1
An example of study qualities (factors), such as form of publication, randomization, and whether the outcomes of studies were adjusted for potential, were used to evaluate the outcome of study

	Peer-Reviewed (%, N)		Randomized (%, N)		Confounder (%, N)	
Study Quality	**Yes**	**No**	**Yes**	**No**	**Yes**	**No**
Source of article						
Journal, thesis	100% (12/12)	0.0% (0/12)	100% (12/12)	0.0% (0/12)	91.7% (11/12)	8.3% (1/12)
Technical bulletin, abstract, reports	0.0% (0/12)	100% (12/12)	33.3% (4/12)	66.7% (8/12)	8.3% (1/12)	91.7% (12/12)
Peer-reviewed						
Yes			100% (12/12)	0.0% (1/12)	84.6% (11/13)	15.4% (2/13)
No			33.3% (4/12)	66.7% (8/12)	8.3% (1/12)	91.7% (11/12)
Randomization						
Yes					70.6% (12/16)	29.4% (4/16)
No					0.0% (0/8)	100% (8/8)

Data from Rabiee and coworkers, 2010,[14] and these study criteria were used in the monensin meta-analysis project.

Table 2
Meta-analysis outcome summary of the effects of monensin on serum/blood metabolic parameters

Variable	Direction of Effect	Percent Change	Significance (*P*)
BHBA	↓	−13.4	.0001
Acetoacetate	↓	14.4	.003
Glucose	↑	3.2	.0001
NEFA	↓	−7.1	.006
Urea	↑	6.2	.0001
AST	↓	Not calculated	.02
Cholesterol	↑	2.6	.076
Insulin	—	17.3	NS
Calcium	—	0.44	NS

Abbreviations: BHBA, beta hydroxybutyrate; NEFA, non-esterified fatty acids.

Meta-regression was used to investigate sources of heterogeneity of the significant responses. This regression method uses the individual effect size for each trial as the outcome and the associated standard error of the effect size as the measure of variance. This approach was conducted by first screening individual variables such as dose, DIM at treatment start, delivery method or diet type in a univariate regression with a liberal P value cutoff of $P = .20$. Some variables such as dose and DIM at treatment start were treated as continuous variables, while other variables were coded as present or absent and were therefore dichotomous. All variables that meet the first screening criteria were then entered into a backward stepwise regression until all variables that remained were statistically significant at $P<.05$.

Tables 2 and **3** illustrate the direction of effect, significance and degree of heterogeneity for metabolic, and production outcomes from the meta-analysis. **Table 4** illustrates the results for the health and reproductive outcomes. In the case of dichotomous outcomes such as disease, results are reported as a relative risk of disease in treated versus control animals.

Table 3
Meta-analysis outcome summary of the effects of monensin on production parameters

Variable	Direction of Effect	Comments	*P* Value
Milk yield	↑	Consistent	<.001
DMI	↓	Consistent	.001
Efficiency	↑	Consistent	.066
Milk fat percentage[a]	↓	Heterogeneous	<.001
Milk protein percentage[b]	↓	Heterogeneous	<.001
Milk lactose percentage	—	No effect	.540
Body condition score	↑	Heterogeneous	.006
Body weight change	↑	Heterogeneous	<.001

[a] Fat yield unchanged BUT heterogeneous.
[b] Protein yield increased, heterogeneous.

Table 4
Meta-analysis outcome summary of the effects of monensin on health

Variable	Relative Risk	Direction of Effect	Comments	*P* Value
Displaced abomasum	0.75	↓	Consistent	.008
Ketosis	0.75	↓	Consistent	.001
Mastitis	0.91	↓	Small effect but consistent	.016
Milk fever	1.11	—	No effect	.309
Calving difficulty	Varies	↑ ↓	Heterogeneous effect	>.10
Retained placenta/metritis				
Sold	0.97	—	No effect	.412
Lame	1.00	—	No effect	.978
First service conception risk	0.97	—	No effect	.283

Graphic representation of the meta-analysis data is a powerful method to assist in evaluating, and interpreting, the results. Forest plots were used to visually display the estimated effect size, 95% confidence interval, and study weights on a single graph. Examples of these graphs are found in **Fig. 1** (acetoacetate) and **Fig. 2** (aspartate aminotransferase [AST]). In these graphs, the box is centered on the mean effect of

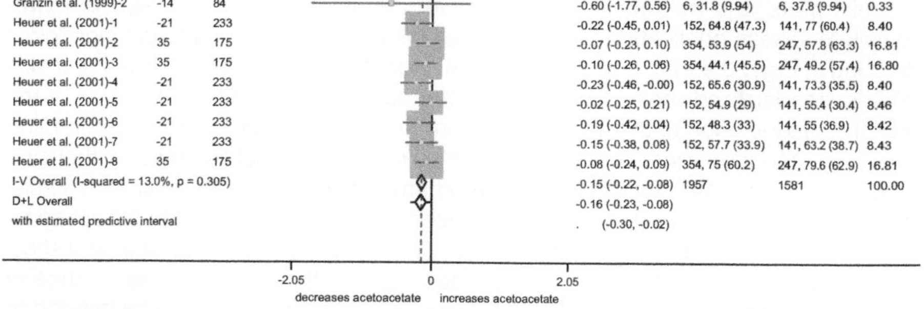

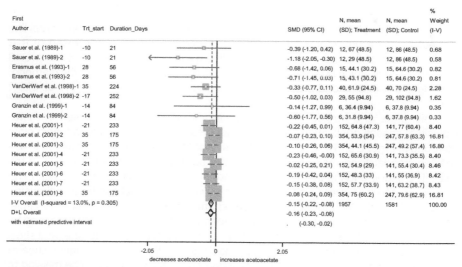

Fig. 1. Forest plot of SMDs and their 95% confidence intervals and weights for individual trials determined from the results of *x* comparisons of cows supplemented with acetoacetate versus other cows. Box sizes are proportional to the inverse variance of the estimates. Summary estimates of treatment effects (*diamonds*) are shown using (1) a fixed effects approach (I-V specifies a fixed effect model using the inverse variance method), (2) a random effects approach (D+L specifies a random effects model using the method of DerSimonian and Laird),[18] and (3) the predicted interval of a future trial, with the estimate of heterogeneity being taken from the inverse variance fixed effect model.

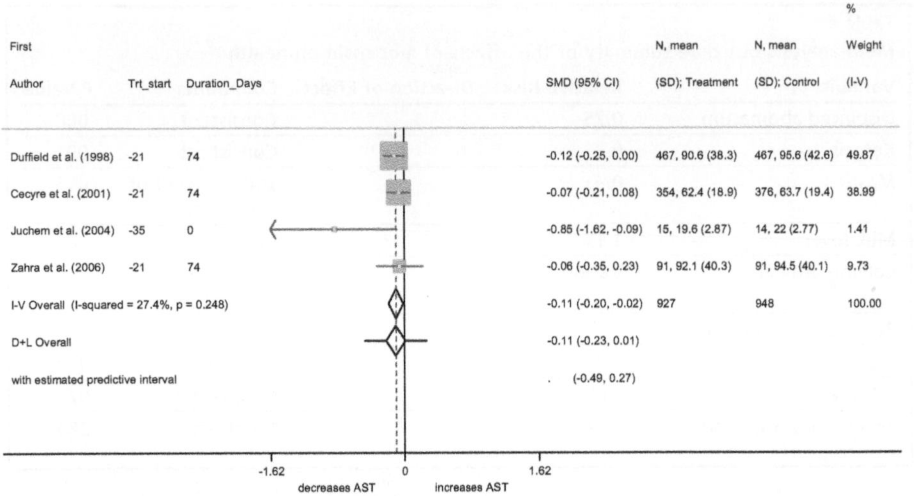

Fig. 2. Forest plot of SMDs and their 95% confidence interval and weights for individual trials determined from the results of 4 comparisons of cows supplemented AST with versus other cows. Box sizes are proportional to the inverse variance of the estimates. Summary estimates of treatment effects (*diamonds*) are shown using (1) a fixed effects approach (I-V specifies a fixed effect model using the inverse variance method), (2) a random effects approach (D+L specifies a random effects model using the method of DerSimonian and Laird),[18] and (3) the predicted interval of a future trial, with the estimate of heterogeneity being taken from the inverse variance fixed effect model.

treatment (monensin) for each study or trial, and the outer edges of the horizontal line connected to the box represent the 95% confidence interval for the mean of that study. The size of the box indicates the relative weighting of the study to the overall mean effect size, which is represented as the dotted vertical line through the diamond. The edges of the diamond provide the 95% confidence interval of the overall effect size.

Funnel plots and contour-enhanced funnel plots are commonly used in meta-analysis to assess publication bias. Two examples of contour-enhanced funnel plots are found in **Figs. 3** and **4**. **Fig. 3** is the funnel plot for DMI, in this case the effect size (SMD is standardized mean difference) is plotted against the standard error of the SMD. The expectation is that larger weighted studies will lie closer to the mean and have lower standard errors. There should, however, be an equal scatter on either side of the SMD, particularly for smaller weighted studies (represented by smaller circle) with greater standard errors. Contour-enhanced funnel plots have been proposed by Peters and coworkers to include contour lines corresponding to the statistical significance ($P = .01, .05, .1$).[16] This approach allows the statistical significance of experiment estimates and areas in which experiments are perceived to be missing to be considered. The contour-enhanced funnel plots may help to differentiate asymmetry caused by publication bias from that due to other factors. For example, if experiments appear to be missing in areas of statistical nonsignificance, then this adds credence to the possibility that the asymmetry is caused by publication bias. Conversely, if the supposed missing studies are in areas of higher statistical significance, this suggests that the observed asymmetry may more likely to be due to factors other than publication bias, such as variable study quality or a failure to

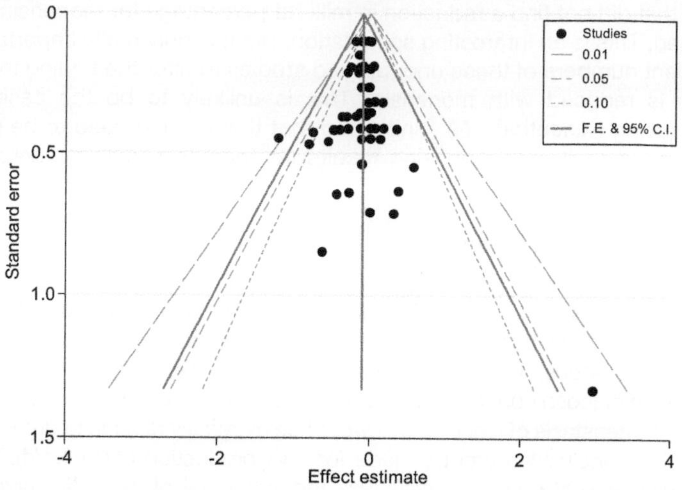

Fig. 3. Contour-enhanced funnel plots of dry matter intake. Levels of significance for studies (•) within the gray broken lines are .01, .05, and .10; FE = fixed effect, 95% CI = 95% confidence interval.

publish findings that were not statistically significant or not be allowed by the reviewers and editors to publish.

For DMI (**Fig. 3**), this is true and there is no evidence of publication bias. However, in **Fig. 4** there is an overrepresentation of smaller studies with higher standard errors and large negative effects on milk fat percentage. This graph suggests that there is the potential for publication bias. Consequently, there may have been small studies

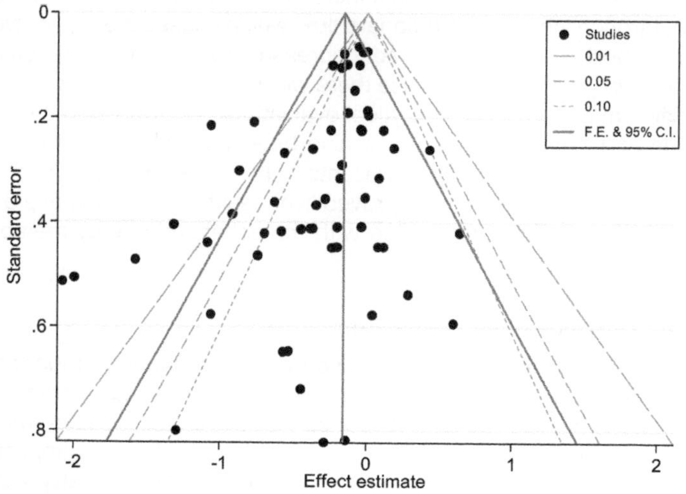

Fig. 4. Contour-enhanced funnel plots of milk fat percentage. Levels of significance for studies (•) within the gray broken lines are .01, .05, and .10; FE = fixed effect, 95% CI = 95% confidence interval.

conducted that did not find a reduction in milk fat percentage for monensin that were not published. This is an interesting speculation, but it is only really important if there were sufficient numbers of these unpublished studies to alter the finding that milk fat percentage is reduced with monensin. This is unlikely to be the case, since a calculation (using Rosenthal's N)[17] indicated that there would need to be more than 137 unpublished trials with opposing results (ie, increased milk fat percentage to reverse the conclusion).

STRENGTH OF META-ANALYSIS

Power to Detect Small Differences

These data illustrate several powerful aspects of how meta-analysis can be used a tool to make better decisions based on evidence gathered. First, there is increased power to detect small differences. The best evidence for this is the conclusion that monensin increases serum glucose concentrations. A change in serum/blood glucose that is highly regulated by homeostasis of just over 3% would be extremely difficult to detect in smaller studies. Similar conclusions can be made for milk production (+0.7 kg/d), DMI (−0.3 kg/d), and incidence of clinical mastitis (9% reduction). All of these findings would be difficult to uncover in most studies because of power limitations. Studies designed to detect such differences with confidence would require several thousand cows to be enrolled. There are considerable advantages in producing consistent databases from studies conducted under many different clinical conditions, rather than large studies conducted in single herds or even at a single research center.

Insights to Other Mechanisms

The meta-analysis findings also help elucidate mechanisms and interrelationships that are affected by monensin. In our metabolic article,[3] we found by testing these effects across the different studies that as non-esterified fatty acids (NEFA) and beta hydroxybutyrate (BHBA) went down, glucose went up; thus, these 3 parameters appear linked. These findings support understandings of the underlying biology[19–21] and previous studies using time-series approaches to evaluate these relationships.[22] The hypothesized causal pathway is that increased energetic precursors are supplied by monensin through increased propionate flux, which causes these positive changes in energy metabolites. The associated decrease in AST concentrations was not presented in the original article because there were only 4 studies (and we decided to require a minimum of 6 for meta-analytical evaluation) that evaluated this parameter. A decrease in AST concentrations could also be linked with the increase in energy available since a lower AST likely represents either lower triglyceride or increased glycogen in the liver,[6] and possibly improved liver health. The finding of a decrease in clinical mastitis may also be associated with the enhanced energy metabolism and improved immune function.[23]

Heterogeneity and Uncovering Mechanisms

Knowing that there is likely to be a response to an intervention is important. Equally important is the consistency of that response from trial to trial. Perhaps the most striking example of heterogeneity of response was the effect found on monensin for milk fat. Although monensin significantly decreases milk fat, this impact is highly variable from trial to trial. This observation led us to look at fatty acids as an outcome and to evaluate diets where possible to examine dietary effects that could help explain this variability. Monensin treatment decreased both de novo fat synthesis (short-chain fatty acids), and saturated fatty acids in milk but increased concentrations of partially hydrogenated fatty acids. This effect is consistent with the effects of biohydrogenation of long-chain unsaturated fats that can cause low milk fat in dairy cows.[24,25]

One of the most substantial advantages of meta-analysis over other forms of review including pooled, weighted analyses of data is the capacity to examine and identify the sources of variation in response to interventions. The use of meta-regression is a particularly valuable development, but subpopulation analysis is also valuable. Our examination of the health data identified a great deal of heterogeneity in retained fetal membrane responses to monensin. Examining responses in populations treated for the whole of the dry period or only part, reduced the variation greatly, and indicated that retained placenta rates tended to be lower in cattle exposed to monensin for only part of the dry period, whereas rates tended to be higher in cattle exposed to monensin for all of the dry period compared to controls.

Meta-Regression Influencers

The use of meta-regression to help explain the heterogeneity of outcomes adds greatly to the strength of meta-analysis. In these studies, we identified greater benefits of monensin for various outcomes for cattle early in lactation and/or cattle fed pasture. In both of these situations, dairy cows could be expected to be in a greater energy deficit and possibly benefit from monensin more. The increased energy supply may also explain the DMI decrease observed, and this effect provides a basis for a milk production efficiency claim for monensin registered in some countries. However, the increased energy supply can be hypothesized to be detrimental as indicated by an increased risk of dystocia or retained placenta when monensin was fed through the entire dry period. However, this effect is usually managed through dietary adjustments. One other important finding from meta-regression was that diets higher in unsaturated fat or lower in fiber showed greater effects in reducing milk fat percentage when monensin was fed.

LIMITATIONS OF META-ANALYSIS

Any meta-analysis is only as good as the articles that it contains. If the criteria for including articles are too inclusive, then the quality of the analysis suffers. However, if the criteria for inclusion are too restrictive, then the analysis suffers from depth and breadth.

Another important limitation is that the meta-regression variables need to be consistently measured across studies as much as this is possible. As an example, it was not possible to examine the effect of monensin on DMI by stage of lactation because too few articles reported this by outcome by stage. Our conclusion that DMI was decreased by monensin is based mostly on full lactation studies. A recent article examined monensin and its effect on DMI in early lactation and reported that it increased DMI in this early lactation phase.[26]

Further, insight is not always available into the underlying biology or is limited in the extent to which this can be investigated. The extent to which underlying mechanisms can be explored depends on the data that are provided. In the case of monensin studies, we were able to explore a metabolic basis for responses.

SUMMARY

Meta-analysis is a powerful tool for making evidence-based decisions for health management and production consultants. Its importance and utility will continue to grow in future years. It is possible that regulatory authorities will make use or allow use of these methods to provide more rigorous evaluation of new technologies and to reduce the costs of developing these technologies and registering these across the world. Meta-analysis will also be increasingly used to provide more rigorous estimates of effect in metabolic and other more basic research studies. In addition, meta-analysis and quantitative literature review will help to encourage better study design and more complete reporting of studies.

REFERENCES

1. Egger M, Davey Smith G, Altman D. Systematic reviews in health care. Meta-analysis in context. London: BMJ Books; 2001.
2. Higgins J, Thompson S, Deeks J, et al. Measuring inconsistency in meta- analyses. Br Med J 2003;327:557–60.
3. Duffield TF, Rabiee AR, Lean IJ. A meta-analysis of the impact of monensin in lactating dairy cattle. Part 3. Health and reproduction. J Dairy Sci 2008;91:2328–41.
4. Duffield TF, Rabiee AR, Lean IJ. A meta-analysis of the impact of monensin in lactating dairy cattle. Part 2. Production effects. J Dairy Sci 2008;91:1347–60.
5. Duffield TF, Rabiee AR, Lean IJ. A meta-analysis of the impact of monensin in lactating dairy cattle. Part 1. Metabolic effects. J Dairy Sci 2008;91:1334–6.
6. Zahra LC, Duffield TF, Leslie KE, et al. Effects of rumen-protected choline and monensin controlled release capsule on milk production and metabolic function of periparturient dairy cows. J Dairy Sci 2006;89:4808–18.
7. Phipps RH, Wilkinson JID, Jonker LJ, et al. Effect of monensin on milk production of Holstein-Friesian dairy cows. J Dairy Sci 2000;83:2789–94.
8. Duffield TF, Sandals D, Leslie KE, et al. Effect of prepartum administration of a monensin controlled release capsule on milk production and milk components in early lactation. J Dairy Sci 1999;82:272–9.
9. Lean IJ, Curtis M, Dyson R, et al. Effects of sodium monensin on reproductive performance of dairy cattle. I. Effects on conception rates, calving-to-conception intervals, calving-to-heat and milk production in dairy cows. Aust Vet J 1994;71: 273–7.
10. Duffield TF, Sandals D, Leslie KE, et al. Effect of prepartum administration of a monensin controlled release capsule on postpartum energy indicators in lactating dairy cattle. J Dairy Sci 1998;81:2354–61.
11. Plaizier JC, Fairfield AM, Azevedo PA, et al. Effects of monensin and stage of lactation on variation of blood metabolites within twenty-four hours in dairy cows. J Dairy Sci 2005;88:3592–602.
12. Stephenson KA, Lean IJ, Hyde ML, et al. Effects of monensin on the metabolism of periparturient dairy cows. J Dairy Sci 1997;80:830–7.
13. Ipharraguerre I, Clark J. Usefulness of ionophores for lactating dairy cows: a review. Anim Feed Sci Technol 2003;106(1-4):39–57.
14. Rabiee AR, Lean IJ, Stevenson MA, et al. Effects of feeding organic trace minerals on milk production and reproductive performance in lactating dairy cows: a meta-analysis. J Dairy Sci 2010;93:4239–51.
15. Sanchez J, Dohoo I, Carrier J, et al. A meta-analysis of the milk-production response after anthelmintic treatment in naturally infected adult dairy cows. Prev Vet Med 2004;63:237–56.
16. Peters JL, Sutton AJ, Jones DR, et al. Contour-enhanced meta-analysis funnel plots help distinguish publication bias from other causes of asymmetry. J. Clin. Epidemiol 2008;61:991–6.
17. Rosenthal R. The "file drawer problem" and tolerance for null results. Psychol B 1979;86:638–41.

18. DerSimonian R, Laird N. Meta-analysis in clinical trials. Control Clin Trials 1986; 7:177–88.
19. Leng RA. Glucose synthesis in ruminants. Adv Vet Sci Comp Med 1970;14, 209–60.
20. Bergman EN. Glucose metabolism in ruminants as related to hypoglycemia and ketosis. Cornell Vet 1973;63:341–82.
21. Lean IJ, Bruss ML, Baldwin RI, et al. Bovine ketosis: a review. Part 2. Biochemistry and prevention. Vet Bull 1992;62:1–14.
22. Lean IJ, Farver TB, Troutt HF, et al. Time series cross-correlation analysis of post-parturient relationships between serum metabolites. J Dairy Sci 1992;75:1891–900.
23. Stephenson KA, Lean IJ, O'Meara TJ. The effect of monensin on the chemotactic function of bovine neutrophils. Aust Vet J 1996;74:315–7.
24. Griinari JM, Dwyer DA, McGuire MA, et al. Trans-octadecenoic acids and milk fat depression in lactating dairy cows. J Dairy Sci 1998;81:1251–61.
25. Bauman DE, Griinari JM. Nutritional regulation of milk fat synthesis. Annu Rev Nutr 2003;23:203–27.
26. Schroeder GF, Strang BD, Shah MA, et al. Effects of increasing levels of monensin on dairy cows in early lactation [abstract] J Dairy Sci 2009;92(E-Suppl 1): 284–5.

Evidence-Based Early Clinical Detection of Emerging Diseases in Food Animals and Zoonoses: Two Cases

Claude Saegerman, DMV, MSc, PhD[a,*], Marie-France Humblet, DMV, MSc, PhD[a], Sarah Rebecca Porter, DMV, MSc, PhD[a], Gina Zanella, DMV, MSc, PhD[b], Ludovic Martinelle, DMV, MSc[a]

KEYWORDS

- Epidemiology • Evidence-based veterinary medicine (EBVM)
- Classification and regression tree analysis
- Early clinical detection • Bovine spongiform encephalopathy
- Bluetongue virus serotype 8 (BTV-8)

Evidence-based veterinary medicine (EBVM) is the application of evidence-based medicine (EBM) to the veterinary field.[1] By definition, it is the conscientious, explicit, and judicious use of the best scientific evidence to inform clinical decisions with a view to improve the clinical outcome at the individual level.[2,3] However, in the veterinary profession, a great deal of time is spent in making diagnostic, therapeutic, and preventive decisions in a complex and uncertain environment where optimal evidence is often lacking.[4]

Medical care is the art of making decisions without adequate information.[5] Medical decision making has been studied extensively and follows a mainstream trend, labeled "rational optimizing."[6] It is usually based on cognitive rational models, such as decision analysis, decision tables, decision trees, and Bayes' theorem.[7–11] When *decision* refers to *diagnosis*, the consideration of the possible causes of a disease, its prevalence, and an initial evaluation of clinical signs will lead to a differential diagnosis about which clinical judgment, informed by evidence clinical data, is exercised.[3]

The authors have nothing to disclose.

[a] Research Unit in Epidemiology and Risk Analysis Applied to Veterinary Sciences (UREAR), Department of Infectious and Parasitic Diseases, Faculty of Veterinary Medicine, University of Liege, B42, Boulevard de Colonster 20, B42, B-4000 Liege, Belgium

[b] Epidemiology Unit, Animal Health Laboratory, ANSES, 23 Avenue du Général-de-Gaulle, F-94706 Maisons-Alfort Cedex, France

* Corresponding author.

E-mail address: Claude.Saegerman@ulg.ac.be

Vet Clin Food Anim 28 (2012) 121–131
doi:10.1016/j.cvfa.2012.01.001 vetfood.theclinics.com
0749-0720/12/$ – see front matter

Diagnosis may involve the choice and interpretation of an appropriate confirmatory diagnostic test.

To detect and identify emerging or rare diseases, a good clinical approach is essential as few biological and epidemiologic data and/or laboratory tests are available. The approach aims at establishing the limits between normality and abnormality as veterinarians cannot relate the clinical signs to those of a known disease or to their experience. These limits should be built on the ability to detect biological variations in physiologic and environmental conditions. The various actors involved in epidemiosurveillance networks (eg, breeders, veterinarians, and slaughterhouse staff) should be prepared for this clinical approach to fulfill their responsibility in health monitoring.[12] Part of this training should develop knowledge of disease biology and epidemiology, and skills in a rigorous, standardized, and evidence-based clinical approach including that of differential diagnosis.[13–16]

Because, with emerging diseases, the implementation of classic EBVM is difficult as a result of few published cases are available and/or accessible via web searches, other options are necessary.

The current report aims to describe a method to improve the early clinical detection of emerging diseases in food animals and zoonoses. This approach is based on the analysis of field clinical observations collected on the first cases suspected of disease using a method called "classification and regression tree" (CART) (Zanella G, Martinelle L, Guyot H, et al. Clinical pattern characterisation of cattle naturally infected by BTV-8. Unpublished data, 2011.).[17,18] Those clinical facts become the only evidence available. Two practical examples are developed to illustrate the feasibility of the method in cattle. Future prospect is also proposed like the implementation of a structured, well-informed and interactive veterinary web clinical data mining platform.

CASE DESCRIPTION

Two examples are developed to illustrate the use of CART analysis for stimulating the early warning of emerging animal diseases. This is a key parameter of health control strategy.[19] CART analysis is a nonlinear and nonparametric model fitted by binary recursive partitioning of data (including clinical signs). Using CART 6.0 software (Salford Systems, San Diego, California), the analysis successively splits the dataset into increasingly homogeneous subsets until it is stratified and meets specified criteria (clinical signs) (**Fig. 1**). Further details about CART are presented in previously original articles or reviews (Zanella G, Martinelle L, Guyot H, et al. Clinical pattern characterisation of cattle naturally infected by BTV-8. Unpublished data, 2011.).[17,18,20]

Case 1: Early Detection of Bovine Spongiform Encephalopathy

Background

Bovine spongiform encephalopathy (BSE) emerged in 1986.[21] It is a neurodegenerative disease characterized by a very long incubation period compared to the life of the host species.[22] BSE started a dramatic chain of events in the United Kingdom and subsequently in other countries.[23] The peak of interest was the discovery of its potential zoonotic character after the first description of a new variant of Creutzfeldt-Jakob disease (*v*CJD) in 1996.[24–26] The presence of clinical signs seems to be linked to the localization and degree of vacuolization of neurons. The main warning signs are psychic disorders (apprehension, temperament change, abnormal ear position, and abnormal behavior), sensory disorders (exaggerated responses to stimuli, excessive licking), as well as postural and locomotion abnormalities (ataxia and tremors). Their

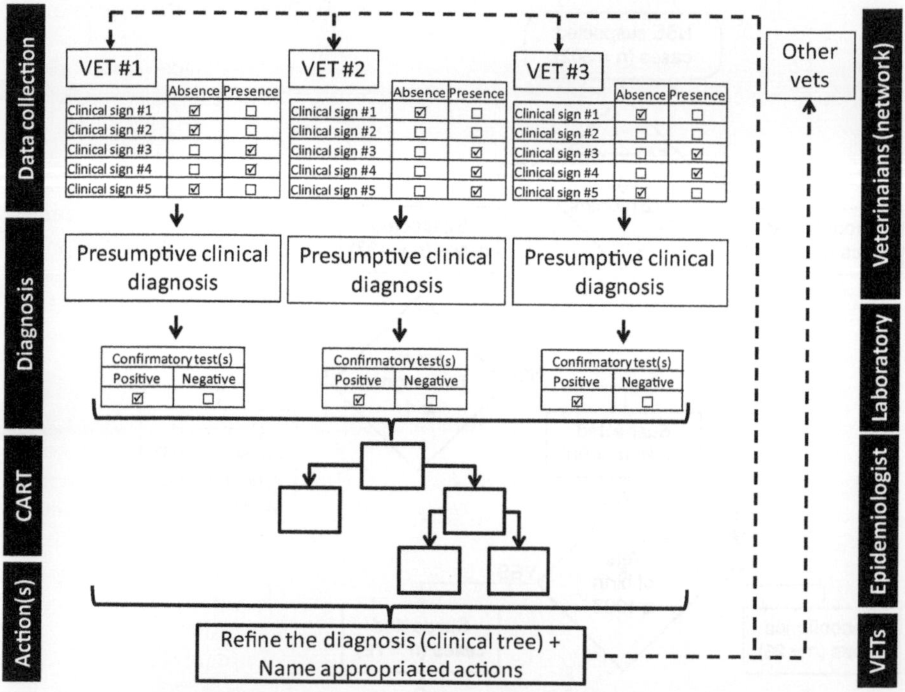

Fig. 1 Flowchart of the CART approach with implication of veterinarians (*left*, process; *right*, actors involved).

identification requires a clinical approach: a thorough veterinary clinical examination of the animal when on a halter and when moving in an uncustomary environment.[16]

Now the evolution of BSE incidence in many European countries is in decline.[27] Because of the favorable BSE epidemiologic situation of most Member States in the European Union, a lowering of control measures, by reducing testing procedure, was recently suggested. However, in such a context, the reporting of clinically suspected cattle by the veterinarians is the most common method for detecting sporadic cases of BSE.[18] The improvement of clinical diagnosis and decision-making remains crucial.

Veterinary data collection

A comparison of clinical patterns captured by veterinarians, consisting of 25 clinical signs, was carried out among BSE cases confirmed in Belgium before October 2002 (N = 30) and 272 suspected cases that were subsequently determined to be histologically, immunohistochemically, and scrapie-associated-fiber negative.[10]

Epidemiological methods and findings

Seasonality in reporting suspected cases was observed, with more cases being reported during wintertime when animals were kept indoors. The median duration of illness was 30 days. Using odds ratio, the 10 most relevant signs of BSE were kicking in the milking parlor, hypersensitivity to touch and/or sound, head shyness, panic-stricken response, reluctance to enter in the milking parlor, abnormal ear movement or carriage, increased alertness behavior, reduced milk yield, teeth grinding, and

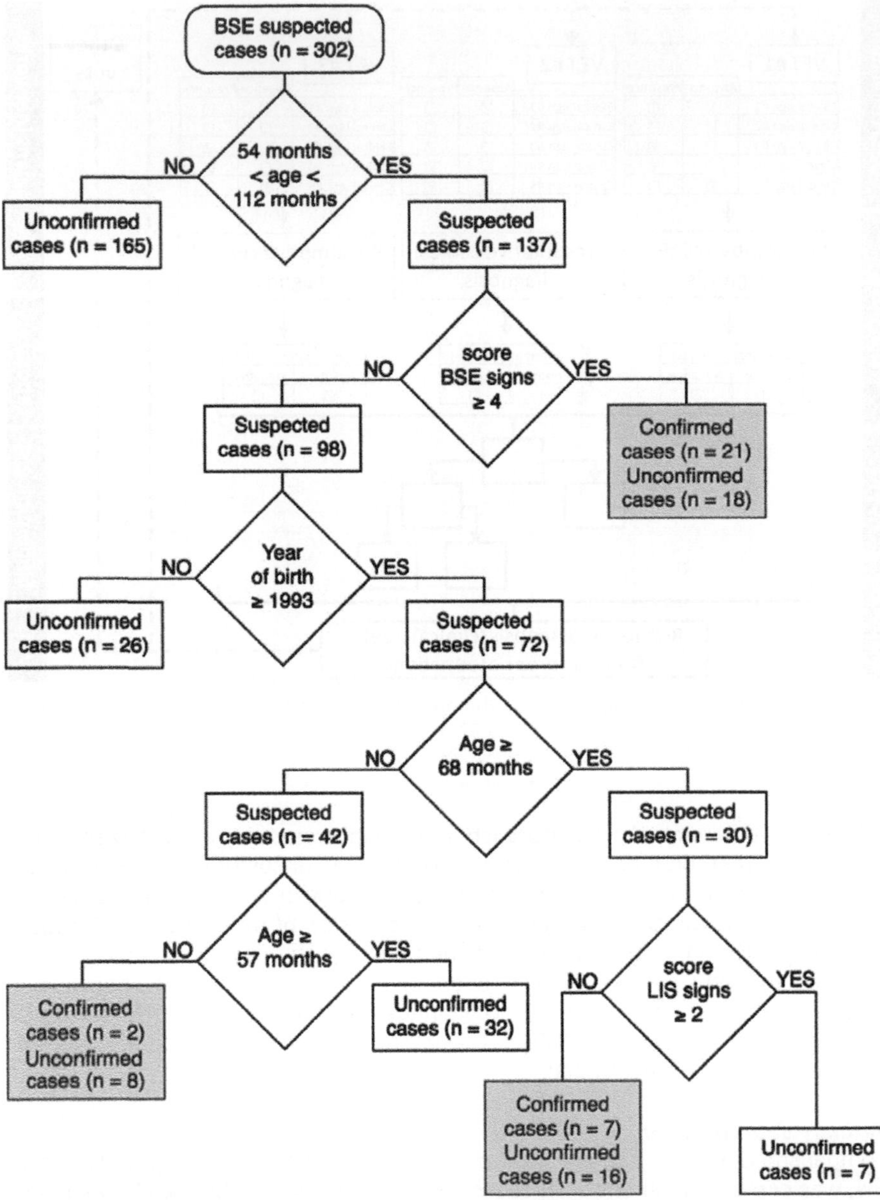

Fig. 2 CART modeling for clinically suspected BSE cases in Belgium.[10] LIS, listeriosis; Score, number of clinical signs that are present.

temperament change. Ataxia did not appear to be a specific sign of BSE. A classification and regression tree was constructed by epidemiologists using the following 4 features: age of the animal, year of birth, number of relevant BSE signs noted, and number of clinical signs typical of listeriosis reported. The model presented a 100% sensitivity and an 85% specificity (**Fig. 2**).

Veterinary significance

The originality of the approach resides in the fact that, first, it involved both veterinarians and epidemiologists. Second, it offered an explorative and interactive tool based of clinical observations (evidence) captured by veterinarians and, then, the results and conclusions are independent of BSE prevalence, through the use of odds ratios. This feature is especially appealing for rare events. A similar decision tree, allowing the distinction between "highly suspected BSE cases" and all other suspected BSE cases, could be applied in other countries, with or without the use of rapid tests. The continued addition of standardized clinical data by veterinarians would permit further improvement of the current model tree, even if the clinical BSE pattern was modified in time. Based on the CART analysis results, veterinarians could more appropriately identify affected cows and retrieve them from the food chain in a public health perspective.

Case Study 2: Early Detection of Bluetongue

Background

Bluetongue (BT) is a noncontagious disease affecting ruminants and is caused by the bluetongue virus (BTV). BTV is transmitted by blood-feeding midges of the genus *Culicoides* (Diptera: *Ceratopogonidae*).[28] A broad spectrum of wild and domestic ruminants can be infected and severe clinical signs are mainly seen in certain breeds of sheep and some *Cervidae* spp.[29,30] The severity of infection depends on various factors, such as species, breed, age, nutritional and immune status of animals, and environmental stresses, as well as the virulence of the BTV strain involved.[31] Although clear differences in virulence of BTV isolates are known, the determinants of virulence are still poorly defined.[31] Clinical manifestations are closely linked to virus-induced vascular injuries and the role of species-specific endothelial cell–derived inflammatory and vasoactive mediators has been highlighted.[32] The European BTV-8 outbreak was characterized by peculiar features.[33] Among these features, a remarkable severity of the lesions in cattle was noticed.[34]

Veterinary data collection

Forty-one cattle from 7 Belgian farms and 2 French farms confirmed as infected with bluetongue virus serotype 8 (BTV-8) were monitored from the onset of clinical signs to describe the disease pattern (Zanella G, Martinelle L, Guyot H, et al. Clinical pattern characterisation of cattle naturally infected by BTV-8. Unpublished data, 2011.). On each visit, a standardized clinical form was filled for each animal by a veterinarian (**Box 1**).[35]

Epidemiological methods and findings

A clinical score was calculated for every week until the end of clinical signs. A CART analysis was conducted by epidemiologists to determine the most important clinical signs every week for the first 7 weeks. The highest scores were recorded within 2 weeks of clinical onset. The first recorded clinical signs were quite obviously visible (conjunctivitis, lesions of nasal mucosa, and nasal discharge). Skin lesions, a drop in milk production, and weight loss appeared later in the course of the disease. A biphasic pattern regarding nasal lesions was noticed: the first peak concerned mainly congestive and ulcerative lesions, whereas the second peak mainly concerned crusty lesions.

Veterinary significance

These results should ensure a more accurate detection of BT in cattle by veterinarians to increase the early detection of emerging diseases (**Table 1**).

Box 1
Bluetongue standardized clinical form for the use in different species[35]

General information: Identification number of the herd; identification number of animal; animal species; breed; sex; date of birth; date of last calving; stage of pregnancy; date of clinical examination; name of clinician

General clinical signs: Hyperthermia; decreased milk production; wasting, emaciation, weight loss; tiredness; edema of head, ears, submandibular region, or the periorbital region; hypertrophied lymph nodes

Clinical signs of skin and annexes: Lesions of the muzzle, lips (congestion > ulcers > necrosis); conjunctivitis, tears, periocular dermatitis; photosensibilization-like lesions; presence of petechiae, contusions, ecchymoses; erythema, inflammation of the skin, crusts; cyanosis of the skin or limbs; skin lesion of the udder, teats or vulva; scrotal skin lesions; wool loss (sheep)

Clinical locomotor signs (musculoarthoskeletal): Incapacity to lift up or prostration; reluctance to move or limited movement; lameness, stiffness of front limbs; lameness, stiffness of hind limbs; edema of coronary bands; swelling of pastern, fetlock, cannon, carpal or hock joint; pododermatitis; contracture of front limbs; contracture of hind limbs; arched back; amyotrophy; torticollis or neck bended

Digestive clinical signs: Loss of appetite; anorexia; difficulties in grasping the food; regurgitation; congestion, erythema of the oral mucosa; ulcerative lesions of the oral mucosa, excoriations; salivation, drooling, foam out of the mouth; edema and/or protrusion of the tongue; cyanosis of the tongue; hemorrhagic stool; diarrhea

Respiratory clinical signs: Ulcerative lesions of the nasal mucosa; purulent nasal discharge; mucous, serous, aqueous nasal discharge; halitosis or bad breath; dyspnea, oral breathing, stridor

Neurologic clinical signs: Apathy, lethargy; generalized weakness, paresis, or paralysis

Reproductive clinical signs: Anestrus; abortion or premature calving; stillbirth; abnormalities of newborns

Duration of evolution: Date of the first clinical signs; comments on the evolution of the disease within the herd

Post-mortem (PM): Has a PM examination been performed? If "yes," please attach a copy of the PM record(s) (with the animals identification mentioned)

Concomitant pathologie(s)

Data from Saegerman C, Mauroy A, Guyot H. Appendix. Bluetongue in ruminants: a standardised clinical report form for the use in different species. In: World Organization for Animal Health and University of Liege, editors. Bluetongue in northern Europe. Paris: 2008. p. 82–7.

DISCUSSION AND SUMMARY

The clinical expression of a disease in an animal depends on several parameters: the nature of the causal agent (dose, virulence),[36] the location of induced lesions,[37] the host (resistance, general condition, immune status), and the environment; some clinical signs may be exacerbated when the environment of the animal is altered.[38,39] The quality of observation plays an essential role and is proportional to the breeders' and veterinarians' level of information, awareness, and training. The intensity of observation is also important, and seems to depend directly on herd size. According to the US National Animal Health Monitoring System (NAHMS), the rate of neurologic problems in breeding females in beef herds, expressed in affected cattle per 1000, doubles when herd size is <100 heads, and is nil when herd size is >300 heads.[40] In addition to these parameters, there is a degree of variability that depends on the

Table 1
Variable importance in CART analysis during the first 7 weeks of cattle naturally infected by BTV-8

	Variable Importance						
Clinical Sign	**Week 1**	**Week 2**	**Week 3**	**Week 4**	**Week 5**	**Week 6**	**Week 7**
Conjunctivitis, lacrimation, periocular dermatitis	100	38		33		100	
Ulcerative lesions of nasal mucosa, crusts	32	100	100	91			76
Mucous, serous, aqueous nasal discharge	26	1		100		28	
Congestion, erythema, redness of buccal mucosa and/or muzzle	21			19		61	
Loss of appetite	18		71	18	3	28	27
Purulent nasal discharge	14			6		13	10
Ulcerative lesions of buccal mucosa, excoriation	11		24	44	0		0
Swelling of coronary bands	7					62	
Skin lesions of udder, teat, or vulva	1			9	32	18	
Swelling of the head, tongue, submaxillary area, jaws			18	22		16	
Lameness or generalized stiffness				2		5	3
Incapacity to stand up, prostration			2	1			3
Anorexia				6			
Tiredness, limited walking				2		47	
Salivation, ptyalism, mouth foam				6		7	
Weight loss			3	62	100	5	41
Arching of back			3				
Muscular atrophy			9	36			
Anoestrus				53		9	5
Milk loss				34	69	78	100
Dyspnea, buccal breathing, loud breathing				5		19	

individual animal and the observer (clinical picture, prepatent phase, and course of the disease). To improve knowledge regarding diseases, especially (re-)emerging animal diseases, it is important (1) to improve awareness, training, and information available for breeders and veterinarians, (2) to use a uniform method for clinical examination by veterinarians, (3) to make more systematic use of confirmatory diagnostic tests, (4) to create sentinel networks of highly motivated breeders and veterinarians, (5) to transcribe the results of observations in a codified and standardized form, regarding both nature and course, (6) to compile and validate existing information by epidemiologists, (7) to enrich a relational database, and (8) to discuss actual experience in a focus group.

In case of early clinical detection of emerging animal diseases, an EBVM approach is difficult to perform. However, an alternative approach based on new structured and harmonized clinical observations (evidence) should be used (standardized clinical form compiled by veterinarians). With 2 practical examples, we demonstrated the usefulness of joint effort involving veterinarians and epidemiologists in CART analysis to improve the early clinical detection of (re-) emerging animal diseases. The strategy is based on analysis of clinical observations (evidences) captured by veterinarians in the field. Selection criteria are based on signs captured by a structured and harmonized clinical form. A presumptive clinical diagnosis performed by veterinarians implies confirmatory diagnostic test(s). Results are analyzed taking into account all clinical signs registered. The CART analysis carried out by epidemiologists allows producing a robust clinical tree that improves the early clinical detection of diseases by any veterinarian who has not faced the considered emerging disease before.

The CART approach is characterized by (1) its exploratory and interactive aspects, (2) its independence from sample size and disease prevalence, which is usually imperfectly known, and (3) its spatiotemporal universality (adaptation is possible when the clinical profile of disease evolves in function of time or region; adaptation is also possible for other diseases). The use of tools to improve the detection of (re-)emergent diseases will lead to more effective veterinary epidemiosurveillance networks. The efficacy of these networks requires regular evaluations together with the elaboration and a continuous follow-up of performance indicators. The recent episodes of both human and animal (re-)emergent diseases have also highlighted the important role of global health information systems. These systems require abilities, resources, collaborative, and coordinated actions of medical and veterinary regulatory authorities.

To improve early clinical detection of (re-)emerging diseases, a future prospect should consist in developing a veterinary structured and informed clinical platform. Whilst some interesting diagnostic support systems for veterinary medicine exist, like the "Consultant" support system from the Cornell College of Veterinary Medicine,[41] no interaction and partition of clinical data are currently available.

Facing the emergence of diseases, the translation of the support system to an interactive platform should be interesting. Involving sentinel veterinarians in this platform is crucial. Veterinarians should be stimulated in a pilot research project to ensure the collection of field clinical data through the filling of structured and harmonized clinical forms. The connection between validated clinical data and results of confirmatory diagnostic tests using CART analysis by epidemiologists permits building useful clinical decision trees to improve the evidence-based early clinical detection of diseases of food-producing animals in the field.

More interactions between veterinarians and epidemiologists should be stimulated in a clinical perspective.

ACKNOWLEDGMENTS

We thank Jean-Michel Vandeweerd for the critical reading of this article.

REFERENCES

1. Cockcroft P, Holmes M. Handbook of evidence-based veterinary medicine. Oxford: Blackwell Publishing; 2003.
2. Sackett DL, Rosenberg WM, Gray JA, et al. Evidence based medicine: what it is and what it isn't. BMJ 1996;312:71–2.
3. Petrie A, Watson P. Additional techniques. In: Statistics for veterinary and animal science, vol. 14. 2nd edition. Edinburgh (UK): Blackwell Science; 2006. p.191–211.
4. Vandeweerd JM, Kirschvink N, Clegg P, et al. Is evidence-based medicine so evident in veterinary research and practice? History, obstacles and perspectives. Vet J 2012;191(1):28–34.
5. Sox HC. Decision-making: a comparison of referral practice and primary care. J Fam Pract 1996;42:155–60.
6. Janis IL, Mann L. Decision making: a psychological analysis of conflict, choice, and commitment. New York: The Free Press; 1977.
7. Eddy DM. Clinical decision making: from theory to practice. Anatomy of a decision. JAMA 1990;263:441–3.
8. Clarke JR, Rosenman DL. A scientific approach to surgical reasoning. Resolving tradeoffs: decision trees and decision analysis. Theor Surg 1991;6:110–5.
9. Cantor SB. Decision analysis: theory and application to medicine. Prim Care 1995; 22:261–70.
10. Saegerman C, Speybroeck N, Roels S, et al. Decision support tools in clinical diagnosis in cows with suspected bovine spongiform encephalopathy. J Clin Microbiol 2004;42:172–8.
11. Abrahantes JC, Aerts M, van Everbroeck B, et al. Classification of sporadic Creutzfeld-Jakob disease based on clinical and neuropathological characteristics. Eur J Epidemiol 2007;22:457–65.
12. Commission Européenne. Règlement 999/2001/CE du 22 mai 2001 du Parlement européen et du Conseil fixant les règles pour la prévention, le contrôle et l'éradication de certaines encéphalopathies spongiformes transmissibles. Journal Officiel de l'Union Européenne 2001;L147:1–40.
13. Stöber M. Symptomatologie différentielle de quelques affections du système nerveux des bovins. Ann Méd Vét 1987;131:401–10.
14. Brown C. Importance des maladies émergentes pour la santé publique et animale et pour les échanges commerciaux. 69ème Session Générale du Comité International de l'Organisation mondiale de la santé animale, 27 mai au 1er juin 2001, Paris, document 69 SG/9 OIE.
15. Schelcher F, Andreoletti O, Cabanie P, et al. Démarche diagnostique dans les maladies nerveuses des bovins. Paris: Proceedings de la Société Française de Buiâtrie; 2001. p. 229–40.
16. Saegerman C, Claes L, Dewaele A, et al. Diagnostic différentiel des troubles à expression nerveuse dans l'espèce bovine en Europe occidentale. Rev Sci Techn Off Int Epiz 2003;22:61–82.
17. Porter RS, Leblond A, Lecollinet S, et al. Clinical diagnosis of West Nile Fever in equids by classification and regression tree analysis and comparative study of clinical appearance in three European countries. Transbound Emerg Dis 2011;58: 197–205.

18. Saegerman C, Porter SR, Humblet M-F. The use of modelling to evaluate and adapt strategies of animal disease control. Rev Sci Tech Off Int Epiz 2011;30:555–69.
19. Merianos A. Surveillance and response to disease emergence. Curr Top Microbiol Immunol 2007;315:477–508.
20. Speybroeck N, Berkvens D, Mfoukou-Ntsakala A, et al. Classification trees versus multinomial models in the analysis of urban farming systems in central Africa. Agri Syst 2004;80:133–49.
21. Wells GAH, Scott AC, Johnson CT, et al. A novel progressive spongiform encephalopathy in cattle. Vet Rec 1987;121:419–20.
22. Lasmézas CI. The transmissible spongiform encephalopathies. Rev Sci Techn Off Int Epiz 2003;22:23–36.
23. Prince MJ, Bailey JA, Barrowman PR, et al. Bovine spongiform encephalopathy. Rev Sci Techn Off Int Epiz 2003;22:37–60.
24. Bruce ME, Will RG, Ironside JW, et al. Transmissions to mice indicate that "new variant" CJD is caused by the BSE agent. Nature 1997;389:498–501.
25. Scott MR, Will R, Ironside J, et al. Compelling transgenetic evidence for transmission of bovine spongiform encephalopathy prions to humans. Proc Natl Acad Sci USA 1999;96:15137–42.
26. Hill AF, Desbrusbais M, Joiner S, et al. The same prion strain causes *v*CJD and BSE. Nature 1997;389:448–50.
27. Saegerman C, Speybroeck N, Vanopdenbosch E, et al. Trends in age-at-detection in bovine spongiform encephalopathy cases: a useful indicator of the epidemic curve. Vet Rec 2006;159:583–7.
28. Mellor PS, Boorman J, Baylis M. Culicoides biting midges: their role as arbovirus vectors. Annu Rev Entomol 2000;45:307–40.
29. Howerth EW, Greene CE, Prestwood AK. Experimentally induced bluetongue virus infection in white-tailed deer: coagulation, clinical pathologic, and gross pathologic changes. Am J Vet Res 1988;49:1906–13.
30. Saegerman C, Bolkaerts B, Baricalla C, et al. The impact of naturally-occurring, trans-placental bluetongue virus serotype-8 infection on reproductive performance in sheep. Vet J 2011;187:72–80.
31. Maclachlan NJ, Drew CP, Darpel KE, et al. The pathology and pathogenesis of bluetongue. J Comp Pathol 2009;141:1–16.
32. DeMaula CD, Leutenegger CM, Bonneau KR, et al. The role of endothelial cell-derived inflammatory and vasoactive mediators in the pathogenesis of bluetongue. Virology 2002;296:330–7.
33. Dal Pozzo F, Saegerman C, Thiry E. Bovine infection with bluetongue virus with special emphasis on European serotype 8. Vet J 2009;182:142–51.
34. Elbers AR, Backx A, Meroc E, et al. Field observations during the bluetongue serotype 8 epidemic in 2006. I. Detection of first outbreaks and clinical signs in sheep and cattle in Belgium, France and the Netherlands. Prev Vet Med 2008;87:21–30.
35. Saegerman C, Mauroy A, Guyot H. Appendix. Bluetongue in ruminants: a standardised clinical report form for the use in different species. In: World Organization for Animal Health and University of Liege, editors Bluetongue in northern Europe. Paris: World Organization for Animal Health; 2008. p. 82–7.
36. Schlech WF. Listeriosis epidemiology, virulence and the significance of contaminated foodstuffs. J Hosp Infect 1991;19:211–24.
37. George LW. Localization and differentiation of neurologic diseases. In: Large animal internal medicine. Smith BP, editor. 2nd edition. St Louis (MO): Mosby-Year Book; 1996. p. 142–70.

38. Kimberlin RH. Bovine spongiform encephalopathy. In: Transmissible spongiform encephalopathies of animals. Rev Sci Tech Off Int Epiz 1992;11:347–90.
39. Saegerman C, Dechamps P, Vanopdenbosch E, et al. Épidémiosurveillance de l'encéphalopathie spongiforme bovine en Belgique: bilan de l'année 1998. Ann Méd Vét 1999;143:423–36.
40. Centers for Epidemiology and Animal Health (CEAH). National Animal Health Monitoring System. Beef'97, part II: Reference of 1997 beef cow-calf health and health management practices. Fort Collins (CO): US Department of Agriculture; 1997.
41. White ME. A diagnostic support system for veterinary medicine. Cornell College of Veterinary Medicine. Available at: www.vet.cornell.edu/consultant/consult.asp. Accessed November 13, 2011.

Evidence-Based Practice? An Evolution Is Necessary for Bovine Practitioners, Teachers, and Researchers

Jean-Michel Vandeweerd, DMV, MS[a,*], Pascal Gustin, DMV, PhD[b], Sébastien Buczinski, Dr Vét, DÉS, MSc[c]

KEYWORDS

- Evidence-based veterinary medicine • Information tool
- Databases • Practitioners

Evidence-based medicine (EBM) is a recent discipline for veterinarians that has largely developed from the concepts promulgated in human medicine.[1] Veterinary pioneers have tried to apply convincingly techniques that are only partially transferable from human to veterinary practice. Several obstacles and difficulties have been identified.[2–5]

THE SITUATION IN 2011

EBM is difficult to practice as veterinarians have only limited time to consult databases and identify relevant scientific information. The task is made even more tedious because not all databases are freely available and search engines are not necessarily adequate for all veterinary disciplines. The amount of literature may be either exhaustive in some areas or extremely limited in others, increasing in both cases the time required to find relevant publications.

For a dairy practitioner, searching peer-reviewed information in MEDLINE on a topic such as "respiratory disease and dairy" leads to a list of 82 references over the past 3 years (assessed on November 24, 2011). The same web-search on "reproduction and dairy" leads to 850 references. If that same veterinarian is not a 100%

The authors have nothing to disclose.
[a] Integrated Veterinary Research Unit - Namur Research Institute for Life Sciences, Department of Veterinary Medicine, Faculty of Sciences, University of Namur, Rue de Bruxelles 61, 5000 Namur, Belgium
[b] Departement of Functionnal Sciences, Faculty of Veterinary Medicine, University of Liège, Liège, Belgium
[c] Département des Sciences Cliniques, Faculté de Médecine Vétérinaire, St-Hyacinthe, Université de Montréal, CP 5000, J2S 7C6 Québec, Canada
* Corresponding author.
E-mail address: jean-michel.vandeweerd@fundp.ac.be

Vet Clin Food Anim 28 (2012) 133–139
doi:10.1016/j.cvfa.2011.12.007 vetfood.theclinics.com
0749-0720/12/$ – see front matter

dairy practitioner but has cow-calf clients who want to know the best vaccination protocol for their calves' preconditioning program, a web-search for "calves' vaccination" displays 124 references over the past 3 years. Using this example and realizing that MEDLINE does not reference the highly assessed periodicals like *Bovine Practitioner* or *Cattle Practice*, one should easily understand that it is not possible to address every clinical question raised every day through an integral evidence-based veterinary medicine (EBVM) approach. A single practitioner would have to stay in the office for many days to assess the information available.

On the other hand, many clinical questions concerning common clinical diseases have not been clearly answered. For example, one should question the efficacy of dexamethasone as an adjunctive tool for treating dairy cows' ketonemia. With the query "dexamethasone and ketonemia and cow and trial," only 1 reference was extracted,[6] in which the dexamethasone was administered alone or with an intravenous dextrose injection. It would appear difficult to answer the initial question since in this study all ketotic cows were treated using corticosteroid drugs.

These various examples illustrate a challenge for bovine practitioners. On the one hand, common questions lead to an impressive amount of information that cannot be assessed easily. On the other hand, common questions have not been specifically addressed and studied. So, EBVM does not appear to be a miraculous way of thinking that will solve every medical or health issue involving cattle or small ruminants.

It is therefore much easier for veterinarians to consult colleagues, specialists, or even the Internet to reach their decision.[7,8] Seeking the best available scientific information becomes a noble objective that most veterinarians are reluctant to reach. Many justifications can therefore easily be used including the lack of proof that EBM helps make better decisions and that experience is far more important than scientific data obtained from research.

Obviously, limited time to keep up to date with the current literature is not an adequate argument against the usefulness of EBM. Searching, accessing, and reading the literature are not just fundamental components of EBM but are fundamental components of being a good veterinary scientist. Assessing the evidence of every clinical decision should be the primary goal of every practitioner in order to give the best level of care for patients as well as to choose the best decision at a population level. It is a question of transparency and accountability. However, even if it was possible for clinicians to dedicate time to obtaining and reading relevant literature, this does not mean that effective EBM is being practiced.

First, available studies may be poorly designed, executed, analyzed, and reported and inadequately peer-reviewed. There are indications that the veterinary literature lacks publications of randomized controlled studies, systematic reviews, and meta-analyses.[2–5] In other words, the practice of EBM necessitates that scientists produce and publish high-standard research with strong levels of evidence.[9] If quality is lacking, quantity is also required to evaluate consistency of results. However, it is difficult for investigators to publish a study that is similar to a previous one, even if it addresses some shortcomings. Peer-reviewed journals do not often allow publication of confirmatory studies. Editors should understand that it is also interesting to repeat studies. It is also sad that scientific data are retained, sometimes legally, for marketing reasons under the cover of confidentiality. A policy of transparency is ethically required. Following specific reported guidelines such as the Reporting Guidelines For Randomized Control Trials (REFLECT) may improve the quality of published studies in reducing the multiple risks of bias induced by poor design of the study.[9]

Second, veterinarians need skills to critically appraise the information that would be available. The language of research, statistics, and scientific methodology is not necessarily understandable by practitioners. We should engage students, academicians, and all veterinary professionals in developing those skills that are necessary to practice EBVM.[10] In addition, the report of material, methods, and results in publications is often confusing and likely too complicated for most veterinary practitioners to take much away from it. We recommend that authors and editors publish accurate and very informative abstracts and summaries in the most intelligible way, considering that the information they contain must not be understandable only by a specialist in the field. Structured abstracts indicating the most important background information, the hypothesis, main study design features, important results, and authors' conclusions would help in a quick assessment of the presented study.

If such informative and clear summaries of high-level publications (like systematic reviews and meta-analyses of strong randomized controlled trials and observational studies) were available on free-access databases, practitioners would be in a position to use modern Internet tools to develop an EBVM approach. This would necessitate that, at the undergraduate level first, then in the course of continuing professional development, they be trained in the basic skills of study design, clinical epidemiology, critical appraisal, techniques of publication, and principles of EBVM. Importantly, EBVM can no longer be the replicate of the classic human EBM and must be defined in its own way, taking into account the context of the veterinary practice.

IS EBVM OUR ONLY CHOICE?

Before looking at possible solutions to develop a practice based on the best available evidence, we could rephrase Dr William Muir, asking whether EBM is our only choice.[2]

Recent data indicate that only a few veterinary surgeons declare that they adopt an EBM approach and consult databases to search the literature in the United States[6] and in Europe.[7] Obviously, this cannot mean that European and American practitioners make poorly informed decisions. These results perhaps illustrate the important role of experience in clinical decisions or the intuitive search of the best evidence.

In addition, there is so far no objective proof that the application of the principles of EBM leads to better practice with healthier animals and more satisfied owners. The advantage of practice that is based on the best available evidence from research is intuitive, as was the use of flecainide in the 1980s against arrhythmias in human patients.[11] This example is often presented in EBVM textbooks to illustrate that the medical community had used, for years, a drug that demonstrated an antiarrhythmic effect on 9 patients.[12] From the conclusion that the drug had antiarrhythmic properties, it was found logical to use that drug on all cardiac patients with arrhythmias. A few years later, randomized controlled studies demonstrated that patients treated with flecainide were twice more likely to die than were those who were not treated with it.[13] From this example, promulgators of EBM state that decisions must be based on scientific proof more than on the logic of a physiopathologic process. Such a statement should also be made about EBVM. The efficacy of the EBVM approach should not be only intuitive but should be proved using the research tools that EBVM itself promulgates (ie, randomized controlled trials, strong observational studies, and systematic reviews).

It is therefore necessary to continue to explore the decision-making process by veterinarians, the role of experience, and the place of peers in education. Obviously, the design of studies that would aim to demonstrate the efficacy of EBVM is extremely challenging. This would necessitate developing measurable outcomes and an accurate EBVM intervention that is well defined, repeatable, and adapted to the veterinary practice.

SUGGESTIONS FOR THE FUTURE

If the veterinary community wants to better understand how they can ensure excellence in their practice and whether an EBVM approach may help, efforts should be made at 3 different levels.

Education

Undergraduate educators should develop skills that are necessary for the practice of EBM: searching the literature in bibliographic databases, rapidly and critically appraising summaries and publications obtained with those databases, and understanding basic concepts of clinical epidemiology referring to the different types of clinical questions that may be asked (regarding etiology, frequency, diagnosis, prognosis, risk, treatment, prevention). Training sessions should prepare students for decision making. They should be able to use a rational approach but also be prepared to act in the real context of practice. This means that they should be trained to make immediate decisions whose effects are not irreversible and that are cost effective; to assess initial decisions and identify weakest points, to obtain colleague or expert opinion, and identify relevant scientific information, that may modify the plan of action; and to explain and justify revision of diagnostic or therapeutic decisions to the client, which is sometimes perceived as confessing a mistake, an excessive risk, a loss of time, or a waste of resource. Importantly, they should be formed to use their background to answer a clinical question and to perceive when it is impossible and when the lack of background necessitates searching the literature to answer what is actually, by definition, a foreground question. Continuing education in EBM is also mandatory, and an effort needs to be made to train the generations of practitioners who have not been exposed to that recent discipline. This could be done via continuing professional development courses and targeted publications in the journals that are most commonly read by practitioners.[14–19] The language of publication could also be a limiting factor, especially for areas of research that are not traditionally performed by researchers publishing in English. The language of publication can limit the depth of systematic reviews if high-quality articles published in a language that is not understood by the researchers have not been included in the literature appraisal.[20]

Due to the increasing amount of available research as previously mentioned, it is impossible that every veterinary student will have learned everything by the end of his or her studies. For these reasons, teaching the EBVM method should be a key component of the veterinary cursus. For example, all these concepts have influenced the teaching of veterinary medicine at the University of Namur and the University of Liège, Belgium. Several implementations have been made at the level of these veterinary schools, as presented in **Table 1**.

Research

There seems to be a consensus throughout the scientific community to develop strategies to improve the level of evidence of the studies and to standardize their reporting.[9] The Evidence Based Veterinary Medicine Association, for example, aims to better organize the emerging research, training, and practice of EBM.

While guidelines to report trials and observational studies were recently published, there is a need to standardize the conduct and publication of systematic reviews.[21] We believe that special attention should be paid to the summary (abstract) of those

Table 1
Implementation of Courses at the Veterinary Schools of Namur and Liège (Belgium)

Year	Course	Description
2	Literature search and use of databases	Students are trained to the use of PubMed and Cab Abstracts in 4 lessons and 2 seminars.
3	Critical appraisal of publications and introduction to EBVM	Four lectures introduce the concept of EBVM, the principles of critical appraisal of publications, the methodology of randomized controlled trials (RCTs) and systematic reviews. This is then applied in 2 seminars: (1) finding and reading abstracts and (2) discussing articles (1 RCT and 1 systematic review).
4	Clinical application of EBVM	Four interactive sessions of 2 hours (voting boxes) referring to 4 clinical questions: (1) how to make a therapeutic decision (antibiotics, for example); (2) how to select a diagnostic test using EBVM; (3) how to use EBVM to avoid litigation; and (4) how to use EBVM principles to evaluate the risk and the prognosis.
5	Multidisciplinary module	This is a module on the mode of problem-based learning (PBL). Over 8 weeks, students work on 14 different problems concerning a wide range of real situations. Several departments work at the design of those problems. Students are trained to make decision and experiment the different phases of the process (quick initial decision, evaluation, more informed decision, legitimization) in a multidisciplinary approach.
6	External rotation and master thesis	The master's thesis requires searching and critical evaluation of the literature. Some theses aim to provide an essay on the decisional process in one complex problem that is encountered by the veterinarian and that students can experience during external rotations.

In this country, 4 universities deliver the bachelor's in veterinary sciences degree (Universities of Namur [FUNDP], Louvain-La-Neuve [UCL], Brussels [ULB] and Liège [ULg]), while only one (ULg) delivers the master's degree. This means that all veterinarians graduate eventually from the same school. These universities are recognized by the European Association of Establishments for Veterinary Education (EAEVE).

studies. A special effort should be made to write informative summaries that are easy for practitioners to understand. A list of the terms and concepts that are used in those reviews should be established so that teachers of EBVM ensure that these are included in their learning objectives.

Editors will be essential actors of the move forward as they could promote systematic reviews and critically appraised topics and be exigent on the quality and accessibility of the summaries. On the other hand, they should be indulgent in accepting confirmatory studies (studies that did not show a significant effect but are of high quality), understanding that they are essential to practice EBM.

Practitioner

Practitioners should be open-minded and willing to take part both in research and in the development of evidence-based practice. We sincerely hope that the current issue of *The Veterinary Clinics of North America* will close the gap that leads most practitioners to view the EBVM practice as an art for the academician but not adapted to the general practice. This necessitates actions in 3 directions.

Private practitioners own a large part of the clinical truth. Every effort should be made to include data from practice in research to increase evidence. This would necessitate implementing and experimenting with data-collecting systems. Ideally, they should be useful to practitioners and optimize recording of clinical data and documentation of the cases. Data retrieval and clinical research would be improved. Applications for practitioners could include improved production of reports and communication with clients and colleagues, data retrieval, or consultation online. This would optimize the time spent by the practitioner in his or her clinical work. Those data-collecting tools are difficult to design, but several prototypes have been reported in the literature.[22–27]

Grounded qualitative study is also important to better understand the role of transmission of experience from veterinarians to their peers and students. Practitioners should also be convinced, and a respectful attitude toward them by academicians would be helpful, that EBVM is not a cookbook that replaces experience. As defined by Sackett and colleagues,[28] evidence-based practice aims to combine clinical judgment and expertise with the best scientific evidence.

Finally, EBVM should be clearly defined in practical terms so that it makes sense for veterinary practitioners, is perceived as being realizable, and, in consequence, stimulates their interest.

A NEW DEFINITION OF EBVM?

In summary of this report and special issue of *Veterinary Clinics of North America: Food Animal Practice,* we suggest a definition of EBVM that takes into account its objectives and practicality. We view it as an information tool that does not replace experience but helps to improve background knowledge and solve clinical foreground questions. It could be defined as the use of accurate, informative and clear summarized information (abstracts) of high level research studies that is obtained quickly via free-access databases available via the Internet and that is provided by a proactive veterinary scientific community in search of transparency, accountability, and evidence.

REFERENCES

1. Cockcroft P, Holmes M. Handbook of evidence-based veterinary medicine. Oxford (UK): Blackwell Publishing; 2003.
2. Muir W. Is evidence-based medicine our only choice? Equine Vet J 2003;35:337–8.
3. Schulz KS, Cook JL, Kapatkin AS, et al. Evidence-based surgery: time for change. Vet Surg 2006;35:697–9.
4. Arlt S, Dicty V, Heuwieser W. Evidence-based medicine in canine reproduction: quality of current available literature. Repro Domest Anim 2010;45:1052–8.
5. Vandeweerd JM, Kirschvink N, Clegg P, et al. Is evidence-based medicine so evident in veterinary research and practice? History, obstacles and perspectives. Vet J 2012;191(1):28–34.
6. Shpigel NY, Chen R, Avidar Y, et al. Use of corticosteroids alone or combined with glucose to treat ketosis in dairy cows. J Am Vet Med Assoc 1996;208:1702–4.
7. Mc Kenzie B. Practitioner survey: Evidence-Based Veterinary Medicine Association. 2010. Available at: http://www.ebvma.org/?q=blog/8. Accessed December 23, 2011.

8. Vandeweerd JM, Vandeweerd S, Gustin C, et al. Understanding the decision-making process by veterinary practitioners: implications on education. J Vet Med Educ.
9. O'Connor AM. Reporting guidelines for primary research: saying what you did. Prev Vet Med 2010;97:144–9.
10. Thomson JU. The building blocks in the professional education process that lead to best practices and quality medicine. J Vet Med Educ 2004;31:6 –8.
11. Anderson JL, Stewart JR, Perry BA, et al. Oral flecainide acetate for the treatment of ventricular arrhythmias. N Engl J Med 1981;305:473–7.
12. Strauss SE, Glasziou P, Richardson WS, et al. Evidence-based medicine: how to practice and teach it, 4th ed. Edinburgh, Churchill Livingstone–Elsevier, 2011.
13. Echt DS, Liebson PR, Mitchell LB, et al. Mortality and morbidity in patients receiving encainide, flecainide, or placebo: the Cardiac Arrhythmia Suppression Trial. N Engl J Med 1991;324:781–8.
14. Vandeweerd JM, Perrin R. Evidence based medicine, la Médecine Factuelle. Prat Vet Eq 2007;156:43–8.
15. Vandeweerd JM. Premiers pas de médecine factuelle: recherche documentaire avec les bases de données. Prat Vet Eq 2009;162:51–6.
16. Vandeweerd JM. La médecine factuelle au quotidien: des suggestions pour les praticiens équins. Prat Vet Eq 2010;166:55–61.
17. Vandeweerd JM, Desbrosse F. Mieux comprendre la validité des tests diagnostiques. Prat Vet Eq 2011;169:55–9.
18. Vandeweerd JM. Fréquence des maladies: notions de prévalence et d'incidence. Prat Vet Eq 2011;170:63–7.
19. Vandeweerd JM. Notion de risque et de pronostic. Prat Vet Eq 2011;171:61–6.
20. Lean IJ, Rabiee AR, Duffield TF, et al. Invited review: use of meta-analysis in animal health and reproduction: methods and applications. J Dairy Sci 2009;92:3545–65.
21. Sargeant JM, O'Connor AM, Gardner IA, et al. The REFLECT statement: reporting guidelines for randomized controlled trials in livestock and food safety: explanation and elaboration. Food Prot 2010;73:579–603.
22. Vandeweerd JM, Davies J, Desbrosse F. A data management system to tackle the challenges of equine practice at the beginning of the XXI century. SIVE Congress 2005, Bologna, Italy.
23. Etherington WG, Kinsel ML, Marsh WE. Options in dairy data management. Can Vet J 1995;36:28–33.
24. Paradis ME, Bouchard E, Scholl DT, et al. Effect of nonclinical Staphylococcus aureus or coagulase-negative staphylococci intramammary infection during the first month of lactation on somatic cell count and milk yield in heifers. J Dairy Sci 2010;93: 2989–97.
25. Sorge US, Kelton DF, Lissemore KD, et al. Evaluation of the Dairy comp305 module "Cow Value" in two Ontario dairy herds. J Dairy Sci 2007;90:5784–97.
26. Mörk M, Lindberg A, Alenius S, et al. Comparison between dairy cow disease incidence in data registered by farmers and in data from a disease-recording system based on veterinary reporting. Prev Vet Med 2009;88:298–307.
27. Corbin MJ, Griffin D. Assessing performance of feedlot operations using epidemiology. Vet Clin North Am Food Anim Pract 2006;22:35–51.
28. Sackett DL, Rosenberg WM, Gray JA, et al. Evidence based medicine: what it is and what it isn't. BMJ 1996;312(7023):71–2.

Index

Note: Page numbers of article titles are in **boldface** type.

Vet Clin Food Anim 28 (2012) 141–147
doi:10.1016/S0749-0720(12)00012-6
vetfood.theclinics.com

I

L

M

N

Printed and bound by CPI Group (UK) Ltd, Croydon, CR0 4YY
03/10/2024
01040460-0011